The Green Lake Library

KETOGENIC
Mediterranean
Diet

The
KETOGENIC
Mediterranean
Diet

A Low-Carb Approach
to the Fresh-and-Delicious,
Heart-Smart Lifestyle

ROBERT SANTOS-PROWSE, MS, RD

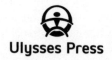

Ulysses Press

Text copyright © 2017 Robert Santos-Prowse. Concept and design copyright © 2017 Ulysses Press and its licensors. All rights reserved. Any unauthorized duplication in whole or in part or dissemination of this edition by any means (including but not limited to photocopying, electronic devices, digital versions, and the Internet) will be prosecuted to the fullest extent of the law.

Published in the United States by:
Ulysses Press
P.O. Box 3440
Berkeley, CA 94703
www.ulyssespress.com

ISBN13: 978-1-61243-641-8
Library of Congress Control Number: 2016950675

Printed in the United States by Kingery Printing Company.
10 9 8 7 6 5 4 3 2

Acquisitions editor: Bridget Thoreson
Managing editor: Claire Chun
Editor: Shayna Keyles
Proofreader: Renee Rutledge
Index: Sayre Van Young
Front cover design: Rebecca Lown
Cover images: salmon © svry/shutterstock.com, olive oil © Taiga/shutterstock.com, vegetables © RTimages/shutterstock.com
Interior design: what!design @ whatweb.com
Production: Jake Flaherty

Distributed by Publishers Group West

To my daughter, Lyra.
May your world be one of never ending wonder.

Contents

Author's Note

I have not always been a nutrition-conscious individual. In fact, in my younger years I was a poster child for how *not* to eat. I grew up in Tennessee in the '80s and '90s, during which time obesity rates increased both at home and throughout the rest of the country. My own growth matched the countrywide climb of obesity very neatly. I gained more and more every year, topping out at 280 pounds by my senior year of high school. I have no memories of ever being at a healthy weight as a child. I remember that every time I went for a check-up with my family doctor, he would tell me and my mother that I needed to "do something about *this*," gesturing to his invisible pot belly.

Body mass index (BMI) is a measure of an individual's height relative to weight, and it is often used as a comparative tool to determine where a person's health fits in with the rest of the population. BMI is judged on a standard spectrum that ranges from underweight to obesity class III. The Centers for Disease Control (CDC) recommends comparing your child's BMI to other children of the same age and height by plotting the child's height and weight on a tabulated chart. From the results, you can place the child within a percentile of growth. My height at that age was fine: I was in the 75th percentile. My weight, however, was literally off the chart. The chart places 210-pound 17-year-olds in the 97th percentile and stops measuring at 230 pounds.

During this time, it was not uncommon for me to drink a six-pack of Dr. Enuf every couple of days or eat an entire pound of Twizzlers in a single sitting. I cannot recall what I knew about nutrition or food at the time, other than that being so overweight did not make high school easy. I do remember that I had a vague idea that my weight was my fault and that I should "do something about it," as the doctor would say.

Occasionally I would decide to get healthy, which usually manifested in one of two ways: First, I would "starve myself" by eating only fresh fruits or salads for as long as I could stand it, which was usually about three days, seeing as I was a teenage boy and all. Alternately, I would try to follow an extreme diet of some sort. I never had great success with any of them because either they were ridiculous, I did not follow them properly, or both.

By the time I was in college and getting my first undergraduate degree, I had managed to lose about 20 pounds by working full time and being a full-time student. I simply had less time to be sedentary. Also, when you have to buy your own food, candy becomes a little bit less of a priority. Even though I was no longer eating my weight in Twizzlers, my diet had not gotten much better. I was still pretty much in the dark about food; after all, my first undergraduate degree was in communications, not nutrition. My diet at this time consisted mainly of Easy Mac with the occasional can of tuna fish dumped into the convenient little plastic cup that is used to serve and prepare Easy Mac. Tired and perpetually hungry, I found it very difficult to resist the comfort of highly processed carbohydrates. I do not think that Kraft intended for Easy Mac to make up the majority of a person's diet, and I sure felt like crap.

It was not until a few years later when I had returned to school to study nutrition that I started to get serious about the science of eating well. I had been working in the print industry but after the strong downturn of 2009 I found myself unemployed. Six months of having my résumé rejected prompted me to go back to school and switch careers. I decided to go into nutrition because, after years of struggling with my weight and watching others do the same, this was a career that would help me finally understand how food really affects the human body. If I could learn how to control my own weight, I was certain that I would be able to help others take back control, as well. In just under five years, I earned a second bachelor's degree—this one in human nutrition— and a master's degree in clinical nutrition. Shortly after that I became a registered dietitian.

Throughout my nutrition education, I experimented with a few dietary and lifestyle patterns and gradually lost another 50 pounds. I was vegetarian for a couple of years and vegan for a while. During my time as a vegan, I also got really into cycling. Yeah, I was *that guy*. My wife and I even tried eating only raw foods for about a week. I was no longer looking to quickly lose weight like when I tried the crash diets in high school; I was more curious about how diet would affect a person's day-to-day experience.

Throughout all of these experiments, I was exercising and trying to eat more sensibly than I had in the past. I wanted to reach a healthy weight, partially since as a dietitian I would be viewed as a nutrition expert, but I was also interested in having the firsthand experience in the things my future clients would be experiencing. I tried the "consistent carbohydrate" diet recommended for diabetics, I did a three-day juice fast, and I followed the post-gastrointestinal surgery recommendations that exclude raw or fibrous foods.

It was this curiosity (and my biochemistry professor) that introduced me to ketosis and the ketogenic diet. In one of our metabolism classes, our professor ran an exercise he called "metabolic accounting" in which we calculated how much molecular energy the body got from processing each of the three major macronutrients: fat, protein, and carbohydrate. I learned that it is much easier for the body to get energy from the digestion of carbohydrate than either protein or fat. This was when I first thought that fat might be a better energy source than carbohydrate for weight management purposes. When I asked my professor about this, he told me about the metabolic state of ketosis.

During my second year of graduate school, I tried the ketogenic diet for the first time and it was a revolutionary experience for me. My weight loss accelerated and I had more energy than I'd had for several years. Since becoming a dietitian, I've continued to eat a ketogenic diet and my weight has stabilized in a healthier range.

When I was approached with the opportunity to write this book, I was excited because it gave me an excuse to further research the long-term benefits of the ketogenic diet and the heart-healthy Mediterranean diet. When combined, these two diets result in an amazingly healthy, delicious, and easy way to eat that leads to fairly effortless weight management, along with a host of other benefits.

With this book, I hope to teach you a little about how your body works to process the food you eat, discuss some of the interesting science behind ketosis, and give you the tools you need to take back your health.

Human metabolism is complicated, fascinating, and not fully understood. While it is not my intention to frame carbohydrates as bad, I believe that there is sufficient evidence to say that most Americans could benefit from some form of carbohydrate restriction. It's true that many healthful diets around the world are based on complex carbohydrates and many people are able to meet the majority of their caloric needs with carbohydrates. However, I propose they are not necessary for health, and that the excessive amount of carbohydrates consumed by followers of a Western diet are at least partially to blame for the rise in obesity, heart disease, and diabetes.

Lastly, a standard but important disclaimer: If you have any disorder of metabolism, especially diabetes, you should personally consult a physician or dietitian (preferably one well-versed in ketosis) before trying the Ketogenic Mediterranean Diet or any other diet. Ketosis can be dangerous for diabetics but does not necessarily have to be. This caveat goes for pregnant women, as well.

Introduction

This book is not a "diet" book. It is not geared toward helping you lose weight. Rather, it is intended to help you transition to a sustainable way of eating that will allow you to be in control of your food choices, eat delicious and filling dishes for every meal, and keep you healthy for years to come—and also result in some weight loss. The ketogenic diet, by its mechanistic nature, results in some loss of body fat. Depending on how much excess energy you have stored as fat on your body, this could be a little or a lot, but I have never met or heard of anyone that did not lose weight while following a ketogenic diet.

The dietary style outlined in this book is a hybrid of two high-profile diets that tend to have devout followers: the ketogenic diet and the Mediterranean diet. Both of them emphasize eating whole foods, both of them have been shown to help control blood pressure and promote a healthy weight, and both of them rely heavily on fat. The combination of these two diets makes perfect sense!

The ketogenic diet is known as a very-low-carbohydrate, moderate protein, and high-fat diet. Such a high-fat diet is perfect for weight loss because fat slows the digestion process and helps you feel full longer than carbohydrates do. Plus, in part because of the rich fat content, the types of foods that fit into a ketogenic diet do not tend to feel like "diet" foods.

The Mediterranean diet probably needs no introduction, as it is hands-down the favorite eating style of clinical and public health professionals. Typically promoted as more of a lifestyle pattern than a diet, the Mediterranean diet includes recommendations for stress management, regular physical activity, and community focus. The diet itself consists of a large amount of fruits and vegetables, whole grains, a moderate amount of meat and dairy, liberal use of olive oil, and a daily glass of red wine. Of course, to fit within a ketogenic diet pattern, the whole grains and most of the fruit will have to be omitted, but we'll get into all of that later.

When I was approached to write this book, I had been following a ketogenic diet for the better part of a year. During that year I lost 30 pounds, experienced a higher and more even level of energy, and began to seriously question much of the dogma claiming that dietary fat is what makes you fat and causes heart disease. The more I read about where that dogma came from and what evidence it was based upon, the less I was convinced that fat is the villain it's made out to be.

As I became convinced that a high-fat, very-low-carbohydrate diet is not only sustainable but also likely preferable for many, I started to think about more than just the weight-loss applications of the ketogenic diet. I began to ask myself what a long-term ketogenic eating pattern would look like. I wanted to craft a diet that includes a large amount of fresh fatty fruits like olives and avocado, low-carbohydrate fruits like tomatoes and artichokes; vegetables; a moderate amount of meat, mostly fish; a moderate amount of dairy; a liberal use of olive oil; and an occasional glass of red wine. Sound familiar? The eating pattern that emerged is the Ketogenic Mediterranean Diet. *The Ketogenic Mediterranean Diet* book combines the easiest, most efficient fat-burning diet with the diet most popular among health professionals for heart health. The result is a way of eating that effortlessly keeps you lean, full of energy, and eating delicious and satisfying meals.

For ease of reading, this book is divided into four sections:

BASIC NUTRITION. Knowledge, particularly in the context of health, is empowerment. I included this section because learning what you are eating and how your body reacts to what you put in it is a crucial part of any healthful lifestyle. You'll also need to understand some of the terms covered in this section for later parts of the book to make sense.

In the basic nutrition section, the major components of food are discussed. You will learn what exactly people are referring to when they use terms like macronutrients and micronutrients. Fats, proteins, and carbohydrates are explained, and we'll explore how the body reacts to each. Particular attention is paid to the various kinds of fats in our food supply, the differences between them, and the health consequences of each type.

Also discussed in this section are the millions of bacteria that live within all of us, collectively referred to as the microbiome. These critters have been shown to have so many beneficial functions for our digestion as well as overall well-being that they are now understood to be a necessary component for good health. What we eat has an effect on which species colonize our gut and how those species behave.

THE KETOGENIC DIET. A discussion of ketosis and the ketogenic diet could easily be an entire book. In fact, many books have been written about this subject (see Resources on page 167 for recommendations). Here, I provide a much shorter overview of the ketogenic diet and how it affects the body.

Researchers are beginning to explore the effects a ketogenic diet may have on a myriad of disease states as well as its potential applications for longevity and cancer prevention. A good portion of this section is spent looking at that research. I'll also cover the regulatory effects that insulin has on blood sugar, because it plays a big part in the effectiveness of the ketogenic diet.

THE MEDITERRANEAN DIET. The foods you eat are not the only important factors of the Mediterranean diet, so in this section I've included discussions on the importance of daily physical activity, stress management, finding a sense of community, and mindful eating. Of course, the nuts and bolts (or in this case, nuts and olives) of the Mediterranean diet are discussed, as well.

KETOGENIC MEDITERRANEAN DIET. This section contains the best of both worlds: the ketogenic and Mediterranean diets melded into one!

By the time you get to this section you should have a good foundation for the information contained within. The diet itself is discussed, as well as the health benefits that you will realize. The lifestyle changes that are a necessary part of The

Ketogenic Mediterranean Diet are covered. Finally, this section is rife with recipes, a meal plan, and tips for success.

After reading this book, you will hopefully have a better understanding of how the food you eat affects your body, a bit more knowledge about just what that food is, and all the tools you will need to completely transform your eating habits for the better.

PART 1
Basic Nutrition

For any of the information in this book to be useful to you, we need to talk about basic nutrition first. This section will be dedicated to food and what your body does with it. Think of this section as a crash course in nutrition, without the tests or tuition. But before we get into the breakdown of the food you should eat, let me take you through the way our bodies break food down.

CHAPTER 1

The Digestive System

When you take a bite of any food, your body immediately begins to break it down in a variety of ways. The most obvious is the mechanical breakdown of food by the teeth. Chewing breaks food into smaller pieces, which increases the surface area available for chemical interaction. And speaking of chemical interaction, a less obvious breakdown is happening in the mouth as you chew.

Saliva, which contains the aptly named enzyme salivary amylase, begins the breakdown of carbohydrates, and the lingual lipase enzyme does the same for fats. As you chew, carbohydrates are already being broken down into simple sugars in your mouth, which is why even the wholest of whole grain breads (the ones that taste like sticks) will begin to taste sweet if you chew them for a few minutes. Proteins just get wet and smashed up. Enzymatic breakdown of proteins does not begin until they reach the stomach.

When you swallow that bite, two things happen: it passes into your esophagus toward your stomach, and we start referring to the ball of mashed food and saliva as a bolus. Bolus may sound strange at first, but it sure trumps "mashed-up food ball." The bolus is pushed toward the stomach by rhythmic muscle contractions of the esophagus called peristalsis. This mechanism works independent of gravity, so even if you stand on your head immediately after eating, the bolus will still make its way to the stomach.

After plopping into the stomach, the bolus gets further digested by the gastric juices waiting there, which are made up of water, hydrochloric acid, and more enzymes. Cells in the lining of the stomach secrete various lipase, amylase, and peptidase (also called protease) enzymes in order to break down fat, carbohydrate, and protein, respectively.

In addition to getting an acid and enzyme bath, the bolus is also being churned continuously. The stomach is literally a bag made of muscles, and those muscles are constantly constricting and relaxing. Depending on the composition of your bolus and your specific physiology, this churning and chemical breakdown continues for anywhere from two and a half to four hours. Very little absorption of nutrients occurs in the stomach, though some water, some alcohol, and many drugs can cross from the stomach into the bloodstream.

Are you comfortable with calling your eaten food a bolus yet? Great, because once the bolus is churned up in the stomach for a bit, we start calling it chyme instead. So far, that's three names for the same bite of food. And there will be more before we're finished. Isn't nutrition fun?

The chyme is gradually let out into the small intestine, which is where most of the actual absorption of nutrients will take place. The small intestine is actually pretty freaking big. In the typical person, it is about 20 to 23 feet long and tightly packed with tiny finger-like projections called villi, which are covered in even smaller projections called microvilli. All of these little fingers increase the surface area of the small intestine by an amazing amount. To repeat the oft-repeated example of just how much surface area we're talking about, if you were to stretch the small intestine smooth it would be able to cover a standard-sized tennis court. I hope that approximation was determined via math and not by physical testing!

Surface area is a big deal in digestion because it allows the nutrients more opportunity to interact with your gut wall and be absorbed. Reduced surface area is why nutrient deficiencies are more common among people suffering from celiac disease, Crohn's disease, or any other issue that damages villi.

Almost all of the available proteins, fats, and digestible carbohydrates in the chyme are absorbed as it moves through the approximately 20 feet of the small intestine. Again, the composition of your food and your specific physiology determine how long this will take. The estimated average transit time is two and a half to three hours.

Anything that makes it to the next and final stage of digestion gets another name. When it passes from the small intestine and into the large intestine, also called the colon, it is referred to as stool or feces. Some people call it poop. That's OK, too.

The large intestine is a little wider, but much shorter, than the small intestine. It is only about five feet long and does not have villi on its interior surface. As the stool travels the length of the large intestine, most of the remaining water is absorbed and the solids are compacted and formed into the shape and consistency that we know as stool. The food you eat and the microbes in your gut play a huge role in the consistency and moisture of your stools.

THE MICROBIOME

Speaking of the bacteria population of the gut, let's take a moment to discuss the microbiome. Microbiome is the term given to the collective bacteria population of your gut. It is estimated that in the average person's colon lining, the number of individual bacteria exceeds 100 trillion. That's up to 10 times the number of cells that make up your actual body.

Though there is still much that we do not understand about the interaction between this community of bacteria and the body, we have evidence of the microbiome playing an important part in our health. In fact, the microbiome is now being called the lost organ because of how important it is to normal bodily function. It seems almost inappropriate to call humans individuals in light of what we now know about the interactions between our bodies and the bacteria in our gut; it is more accurate to say that we are all synergistic communities.

So far, we know that the microbiome plays an important role in immunity, weight regulation, mood regulation, and possibly even longevity. Unfortunately, we do not yet know the exact nature of that role.

We do know that the human bacterial population is made up of thousands of different species, each with its own behavior and effect. All of these bacteria need food to flourish, and many species seem to prefer fiber as their food. Because all fiber comes from carbohydrates and a ketogenic diet is very low carbohydrate, one of the concerns about ketogenic eating is that it will negatively affect the composition of the microbiome. Fortunately, a ketogenic diet, particularly the Ketogenic Mediterranean Diet, does not have to be a low-fiber diet.

HOW WE ACTUALLY GET ENERGY

The above overview of the digestive system helps you understand, from a systematic perspective, what happens in your body after you eat. To take it one step further, let's talk about what your body does with the food once it is small enough to pass from your digestive system into the rest of the body, where it can be used by individual cells.

Most of what we eat is broken down into its component parts and either run through cellular pathways to extract the chemical energy (I'll refer to energy being "burned" from now on) or used to build other things. Imagine, if you will, that you have a sandwich made from Legos. You can take the Lego-wich apart and have a pile of pieces to work with. You could assemble them back together as a rocket or a house or, as I did as a child, a multicolored nothing that you are proud of anyway. Alternately, you can eat these Legos and use them for energy. Finally, you could put the blocks in a bag and save them for later.

These are the options your body faces constantly. Most of what you give it can be torn apart and put back together differently, burned for energy, or stored for later use. Which action your body takes depends on many factors, like its current energy needs and the food available at the time.

Now that we've taken a journey through the digestive system, with brief detours into the microbiome and food made of Legos, we will explore the composition of food and how it is classified. Chapter 2 will be dedicated to the macronutrients: fat, protein, carbohydrates, and alcohol. Chapter 3 is about the micronutrients, vitamins, and minerals, and which are most relevant to the Ketogenic Mediterranean Diet.

CHAPTER 2

The Macronutrients

It seems like there are a million different ways to classify food—calorie content, organic status, processing level, glycemic load, pH influence, allergen content, and so on. This chapter covers macronutrient classifications, one of the most basic but most useful ways to break food into categories. Macronutrients are defined as chemical compounds that provide energy when consumed. There are three major macronutrients: protein, fat, and carbohydrate. We'll also include alcohol as a macronutrient, because it can be burned for energy. Almost all foods contain a combination of protein, fat, and carbohydrate, but for the sake of simplicity, we often lump them into categories based on whichever macronutrient makes up the greatest proportion of their composition.

PROTEIN

Protein is used to build and maintain muscle and other bodily tissues. It is also used to make hormones, immunoglobulins for the immune system, lipoproteins for substance transport, and hemoglobin in the blood. In fact, almost every part of your body needs protein to function properly and is at least partially made of protein. It can also be used as an energy source either on its own or after being converted into glucose.

All protein is made up of smaller units called amino acids. There are over 500 amino acids that have been identified in nature, but we only eat about 20 of them, and in most instances, we only *need* to eat nine of them. These nine are called essential amino acids because our bodies cannot make them and we have to get them through food for optimal health. There are few situations in which some of the other 11 amino acids need to be supplemented through diet, too. In those cases, we call the amino acids conditionally essential.

The protein that you eat is made up of long chains of these different amino acids. Your body takes those chains apart and then uses the individual amino acids to build other things, or it burns them to get energy. As a rule of thumb, protein provides four calories per gram.

Protein can come from animal-based sources or plant-based sources. Just about every animal product is a good source of protein. Beef, chicken, pork, fish, egg, most cheeses, yogurt, and milk all contain good amounts of protein. The exceptions include things like butter and cream, which are mostly fat. There are also many great plant-based sources of protein that we will be using in the Ketogenic Mediterranean Diet. Nuts and seeds are both fantastic sources of protein that are low enough in carbohydrates to fit our needs. Though beans are good sources of plant-based protein, most are too high in carbohydrates, so the only bean we will be including on a regular basis in our diet is the soybean. Don't worry; we'll get into all of that in later chapters.

Functionally, there is a little bit of difference between plant- and animal-based proteins. Animal-based protein tends to have a more complete mix of those essential amino acids we discussed; that is to say, a single source of animal-based protein is likely to be a good source of all nine of the essential amino acids. Plant sources tend to have an adequate amount of a few of the essentials, but usually not all of them. That's why it is even more important for vegetarians to eat a variety of foods.

Protein is the most import of the macronutrients because it is used for so many essential things in the body. Most people that are in developed nations have absolutely no issue getting enough protein for bodily maintenance and development.

The recommended daily allowance (RDA) for protein, which is a metric set by the Institute of Medicine, is 0.8 grams per kilogram of body weight. For a 160-pound sedentary male, this equates to about 58 grams of protein per day, and for a 140-pound sedentary female, about 51 grams. These amounts should be regarded as minimum daily levels for healthy people and, as you will know if you have ever tracked your food intake, it is very easy to reach this level of protein intake. Larger individuals, people with a lot of muscle, or people who are attempting to build muscle will need to eat more protein to maintain and build muscle mass.

There is currently no recommendation for maximum daily protein intake but there is such a thing as protein toxicity, which happens if you consume more protein than the body can process. Because nitrogen, a byproduct of protein metabolism, can be detrimental in high quantities, the liver must process it into a form that the kidneys can safely excrete. There is evidence that there is an upper limit to how much nitrogen the liver is able to process at a time. However, this limit appears to be somewhere around three and a half to four and a half grams per kilogram, meaning it would be difficult to reach intake levels this high unless you were intentional about it. That equates to 280 to 360 grams per day for an average male.

From a ketogenic perspective, I recommend keeping protein intake between one and a half to two grams per kilogram because of the body's ability to convert excess protein into glucose. Too much glucose in the blood will inhibit ketone production and so, theoretically, excessive protein intake would be counterproductive to a ketogenic diet. I'll discuss this in more detail in Chapter 4: Mechanics of the Ketogenic Diet.

FAT

Fat has by far been the most polarizing nutrient in the United States over the past 40 years. Starting in 1977, Americans were told to eat less fat because it would potentially make their arteries harden and eventually lead to heart failure. Since then, many books have been written about how these recommendations are misguided and not scientifically based.

Fat is an essential nutrient for several reasons. Like the other essential nutrients, your body cannot make all the fat that it needs. Second, like protein, it is directly a part of many of your body's structures. Fat is incorporated into the structure of all of your organs, but your brain, which is made of around 60 percent fat, is actually the fattiest—so I guess in a way, we are all fat heads. Fat is also the primary component of the protective coating of nerve endings called myelin. Without these protective coatings, nerve signaling cannot function properly.

Hormones are another component of the body that would not be possible without fatty acids, which are the building blocks of fats. Many of the hormones in our body are referred to as lipid-derived because they are made from fats. On a cellular level, fat is even more important. All cells have an outer wall composed of a lipid bilayer that allows them to maintain separation from extracellular materials. Without these lipid bilayers, there would be no life at all. *That's* what I call essential.

Additionally, we require fats to absorb certain nutrients. The vitamins A, D, E, and K are referred to as fat-soluble vitamins because they literally cannot be absorbed without first being surrounded by fat. Unlike the other vitamins, which are water-soluble, these four can be stored in the body's fat tissues.

Fat is also an important source of energy for the body, and for maybe as much as two thirds of the population, it should be the most important and preferred fuel source. Fat provides nine calories per gram, over twice what protein and carbohydrates provide. It is also the only of the three major macronutrients that does not induce an insulin response in the body. This, as you will see in later chapters, is a very important feature of fat metabolism for long-term optimal health. Your body understands the value of fat as fuel so well that it utilizes fat as long-term energy storage.

The fat tissue on our bodies is made up of adipocytes packed full of triglycerides. Triglycerides are the body's long-term storage solution for energy that is not immediately needed.

Certainly some of our body fat comes from dietary fat, but for most people eating the Standard American Diet (SAD), much of the fat tissue on their bodies is actually excess carbohydrate that the body has converted into fat. That's right—excessive carbohydrate is easily turned into body fat.

Structurally, fat is fairly simple: it is a long chain of carbon atoms bound together with hydrogen atoms attached to the top and bottom of each carbon. If every available spot along the chain is filled, we call this saturation, and those saturated chains are called saturated fats. Any spot along this carbon chain that is not bound by two hydrogen atoms is called an unsaturation point. Fats with only one unsaturation point are called monounsaturated fats and fats that have more than one are referred to as polyunsaturated fats. Makes sense, right?

If you've ever wondered about why omega-3 fats and omega-6 fats (also known as fatty acids, or n- fats) are named that way, well, it is also because of their structure. Fats are named by where their first unsaturation point occurs. So on omega-3 fats, the first carbon that is not paired with hydrogen atoms is the third. This does not give any indication as to how many saturation points there are, just where the first one occurs.

And finally, what is a trans fat? For our purposes, a trans fat forms when an unsaturated fat has been artificially converted into a saturated fat by the addition of hydrogen atoms. That's why anything that has partially hydrogenated oils will contain trans fat. Changing a fat from unsaturated to saturated is desirable from an industry perspective because it allows for longer shelf life. However, trans fats are undesirable from a health perspective because the US Food and Drug Administration (FDA) believes that these artificially saturated fats are associated with a greatly increased risk of heart disease. They recommend avoiding trans fats altogether and have banned their use in foods, but there are always loopholes that the food industry is very adept at exploiting. Even with the ban, it is a good idea to read labels and avoid products containing partially or fully hydrogenated fats. There are such things as naturally occurring trans fats that are found in meats and dairy products, but these have not been associated with the heart disease risk that man-made trans fats seem to increase.

That's a basic overview of fats, but let's go a little deeper into the functional and nutritional properties of saturated, mono-unsaturated, and polyunsaturated fats before moving on to carbohydrates, since these distinctions are such hot topics in the health community and will be very important to our discussion of the Ketogenic Mediterranean Diet.

Although fats are never 100 percent saturated or unsaturated but always a mix, we usually refer to them by whatever percentage is highest. I'll be using this convention for the rest of this section.

SATURATED FAT

You can typically tell if a fat is saturated if it remains solid at room temperature. Most of the sources of saturated fat are animal in nature. Butter, lard, and the fats found in meats and cheeses are saturated fats. The fats found in plants are mono or polyunsaturated fat with two notable exceptions: coconut and red palm. The oils from both of these tropical plants consist of mostly saturated fats and will stay solid at room temperature. If you look at the ingredients in stores, you will note that red palm oil is replacing many of the partially hydrogenated oils that were used prior to the ban.

Alarms will likely be going off in your head about now to the tune of "SATURATED FAT CAUSES HEART DISEASE!"

I don't blame you. The government has been pushing that line hard for the past 40 years in the United States. The only problem is that the recommendations to avoid saturated fat were not based on sound science, and the practice of avoiding saturated fats has not been doing a great job of making us healthier. I assume that because you picked up a book with the word "ketogenic" in its title, you are already at least questioning these recommendations.

I'll calm your alarms now. I do not recommend that a person eating the Standard American Diet consume a high saturated fat content. However, if you are following a ketogenic diet and your metabolism has adjusted to use fat as its primary fuel source, saturated fats are perfectly acceptable. In fact the specific type of saturated fat found in coconut, medium-chain triglycerides, actually promotes the production of ketones and can be a wonderfully healthful addition to a ketogenic diet plan.

MONOUNSATURATED FAT

Monounsaturated fats are as loved by health professionals as saturated fats are hated. Monounsaturated fats will be liquid at room temperature but will get solid when chilled. Good sources of monounsaturated fats are nuts, seeds, and fatty fruits such as olives and avocados. The Ketogenic Mediterranean Diet abounds with sources of these fats. In people eating the SAD diet, replacing saturated fats with mono or polyunsaturated fats is thought to lower LDL ("bad" cholesterol) and raise HDL ("good" cholesterol).

POLYUNSATURATED FATS

Polyunsaturated fats are those with two or more of the unsaturation points we discussed above. Polyunsaturated fats, when consumed in moderation, are also well loved by the health establishment because of the associations found between these fats and reduced risk of chronic diseases. Omega-3 and omega-6 fats are both polyunsaturated. The issue for many Americans is that they get way too much of the n-6 fats and not enough of the n-3s. Let's take a closer look at those.

OMEGA-6 FATTY ACIDS. This subclass of polyunsaturated fats is found abundantly in the American diet in vegetable oils like soy, corn, and safflower oils. These oils are commonly used in the industrial food supply and are found in many processed foods. Omega-6 fatty acids have been shown to either promote or inhibit inflammation, depending on the concentration.

OMEGA-3 FATTY ACIDS. These are harder to find in our food supply, but their health benefits are less ambiguous: they are almost universally understood to be beneficial. Omega-3 fatty acids are found most abundantly in marine foods like fish, fish oils, and algae; and in certain nuts and seeds like walnuts, flaxseeds, and chia seeds. The most beneficial omega-3 fatty acids are docosahexaenoic acid (DHA) and eicosapentaenoic acid (EPA), which are found almost exclusively in algae and marine life. The omega-3 fatty acid found in nuts and seeds is typically alpha-linolenic acid (ALA) and must be converted in the body to DHA or EPA. This conversion is difficult because the pathway used for this conversion is shared by n-6 fatty acids, resulting in a slow process, particularly when n-6 fats are abundant. That's why it is best to eat DHA and EPA directly.

OMEGA-6 TO OMEGA-3 RATIO. Given that both of these fats appear to be healthy in the right quantities, it looks like the ratio of n-6 to n-3 is the important factor to health outcomes. Prior to industrialization of society, their ratio was somewhere in the range of 4:1 and 1:4, depending on the availability of seafood. This is close to the theoretically ideal ratio of 1:1. In people eating the SAD diet, this ratio has been measured at somewhere from 15:1 to 17:1.

CARBOHYDRATES

Oh, carbohydrates. They are unique among the macronutrients. Unlike fats and proteins, carbohydrates are *not* a required nutrient. Let me say that again: Humans do not need to consume any quantity of carbohydrates for optimal health. *None.* Our bodies can make the very limited amount of glucose that we need, so long as we consume adequate protein. Carbohydrates are also the only macronutrient that stimulates the release of serotonin, one of the hormones associated with pleasure and happiness, upon consumption. In this way, carbohydrates can become addictive, and I have witnessed individuals experience the symptoms of withdrawal when initially restricting carbohydrates in their diet. Finally, carbohydrates are unique in the way that the body reacts to them.

Excessive carbohydrate intake (more than 20 to 50 grams per day, depending on the individual) promotes the release of insulin into the bloodstream like no other nutrient. Insulin is a hormone with many jobs in the body, one of which is to take glucose out of the bloodstream and begin the process of turning it into stored fat in the body.

Carbohydrates come in a few different forms. In their simplest forms, carbohydrates are called monosaccharides, with *mono* meaning single and *saccharide* meaning sugar. The monosaccharides often found in the foods we eat are glucose, fructose, and galactose. These three are combined in several combinations to make the sugars we are used to seeing.

SUGAR	COMBINATION
Lactose (dairy sugar)	Glucose + Galactose
Maltose (malt sugar)	Glucose + Glucose
Sucrose (table sugar)	Glucose + Fructose

There has been much discussion recently regarding how the body reacts to glucose versus fructose, but it is honestly not that important if you are considering the damaging effects of carbohydrates as a whole. Cigarettes and chewing tobacco do different things to the body for sure, but both are detrimental to your health, provide no significant benefit, and should be avoided. The same is true of dietary glucose and fructose.

Because we are discussing a dietary pattern that involves severe restriction of all carbohydrates, I don't think it will be useful to discuss them in depth. We just need to understand that as a category, "carbohydrates" include simple sugars such as glucose and fructose, which are important from a metabolic perspective; disaccharides, through which these simple sugars are usually delivered; starch, which is a long chain of glucose found in plants; and fiber, which also consists of polysaccharides, long chains of monosaccharides bound together, but are composed of different saccharides that we cannot digest. Let's talk about fiber in a little more detail because it can be very useful when following a ketogenic diet.

DIETARY FIBER

The fiber that we eat comes in two forms: soluble and insoluble. We cannot digest either one, and the microbes living in our large intestine (the gut microbiome) are responsible for any breakdown that occurs. Fiber is of special interest to us in the ketogenic community because we can subtract the amount of fiber a food contains, in grams, from the amount of total carbohydrate to get an idea of how many actual grams of insulin-inducing carbohydrates exist in a food. Of course, this calculation is not perfect, and you will need to experiment to see how careful you need to be using this "net carbs" method, but it can definitely broaden the range of foods you will be able to include.

SOLUBLE FIBER. Soluble fiber dissolves in water and is relatively easy for the bacteria in your gut to ferment. One of the byproducts of that fermentation are short-chain fatty acids. Short-chain fatty acids are metabolized primarily by the cells in the colon and are important for gut health. Other than being fermented, soluble fiber is useful for producing regular and consistent stool movements. As it forms a gel when moving through your colon, soluble fiber adds bulk to your stool and helps prevent both constipation and diarrhea.

INSOLUBLE FIBER. Insoluble fiber does not dissolve in water and moves through the digestive tract mostly untouched. It can also be a good source of food for the microbiome and is considered a prebiotic. Those with gastrointestinal regularity issues cherish insoluble fiber because it fairly reliably adds bulk and regularity to stools. While both soluble and insoluble fiber help with all things poop related, insoluble fiber is regarded as the more helpful of the two.

ALCOHOL

Alcohol is technically a macronutrient because it provides energy, but it should not be considered a useful addition to your diet. From an energy perspective, alcohol provides seven calories per gram. While it is fine to include some alcohol in your Ketogenic Mediterranean Diet, you shouldn't include a great deal. Alcohol is technically a poison that must be metabolized by the liver and filtered out of the blood by the kidneys.

People who are in ketosis are already retaining less water than those eating a carbohydrate-heavy diet. Because alcohol toxicity (which occasionally shows up as a hangover) is partially linked to dehydration, it is much more common to suffer from the negative effects of alcohol overconsumption while in ketosis. Trust me, you'll want to keep your alcohol consumption reasonable. That means only one or two servings of alcohol (five ounces of wine, one ounce of a distilled alcohol like whiskey or vodka, or twelve ounces of beer) per day.

Other than the negative reinforcement of feeling terrible the next day, it should be easy to stick to these amounts because alcoholic beverages also tend to have a moderate carbohydrate content. Alcohol itself is not a carbohydrate, but beverages like wine and beer with lower alcohol contents still contain much of the original carbohydrate content from the food that they were made from (grapes for wine, and grains like wheat or barely for beer).

CHAPTER 3

The Micronutrients

Micronutrients are chemical elements required in small amounts for normal growth and function in the human body. The micronutrients include all of the vitamins and minerals. There are many, many micronutrients and it is not necessary for us to discuss all of them here—plus, you'd be really bored if I did. Instead, I'll just give you an overview of the vitamins and minerals and why they are specifically relevant to our Ketogenic Mediterranean Diet.

VITAMINS

Vitamins are divided into two categories based on what they will dissolve in. Water-soluble vitamins can be dissolved in water, while fat-soluble vitamins require some fatty acids to be absorbed.

There are no specific vitamin requirements for an individual in ketosis compared to someone eating a carbohydrate-heavy diet. Further, a person following a well-planned ketogenic diet will not be lacking any vitamins in sufficient quantities. In fact, the Ketogenic Mediterranean Diet is so vitamin-rich that by adopting that lifestyle, you will likely be getting a more complete mix of vitamins and minerals than you were before.

WATER-SOLUBLE VITAMINS. Water-soluble vitamins play many important roles in the body, specifically when it comes to the transfer and production of energy. Thiamin, riboflavin, niacin, pantothenic acid, and biotin in particular help with the breakdown of nutrients and their conversion to usable energy. Vitamins C, B6, and B12 all help build structures. While these vitamins are not incorporated into the cells they help build, they are necessary for their construction.

- biotin (B7)
- folic acid (B9, or folate)
- niacin (B3)
- panthothenic acid (B5)
- riboflavin (B2)
- thiamin (B)
- vitamin B6
- vitamin B12
- vitamin C

FAT-SOLUBLE VITAMINS. Some of the major functions of the fat-soluble vitamins include keeping your tissues in good repair, protecting your vision, acting as antioxidants, and building bones. Vitamins D and E are also thought to play some role in mood regulation, and vitamin K is a major player in blood clotting. It is important to note that all of the vitamins are almost certainly involved in many more processes than we currently understand.

Because they are able to build up over time, it is possible for vitamins A, E, and K to cause damage if they are chronically overconsumed. So far, there have not been any negative consequences associated with large amounts of vitamin D consumption. This is likely because vitamin D is not actually a vitamin; rather, it is hormone that we just call a vitamin.

- ▸ vitamin A
- ▸ vitamin E
- ▸ vitamin D
- ▸ vitamin K

MINERALS

Unlike vitamins, minerals *are* incorporated into the body's structures. Most of the bone matrix is made up of the minerals calcium and phosphorus. Minerals also perform a huge variety of other functions in the body. Basically, if you can think of something that your body does, you need at least one mineral to make it happen. Dietary minerals can be divided into two categories, major and trace, based upon the amount of the mineral found in the body.

Also unlike with vitamins, there are additional mineral requirements for those eating a ketogenic diet. Ketosis stimulates the kidney to shed sodium at a faster rate. Sodium levels in the body drive potassium levels, because the body is constantly trying to keep levels of sodium and potassium at a certain ratio. Because sodium is not found in high concentrations naturally, you will likely need to consciously increase your sodium intake on the Ketogenic Mediterranean Diet. We'll discuss ways to do that in later chapters.

MAJOR MINERALS. Compared to the vitamins and trace minerals, we have quite a lot of the major minerals in our bodies. Most of them are involved in some way with fluid balance or structure stabilization. They are also important for electrical signaling and cell transfer.

- calcium
- chloride
- magnesium
- phosphorus
- potassium
- sodium
- sulfur

TRACE MINERALS. When I say trace, I really mean it. All of the trace minerals in your body could easily fit inside a thimble. Though there is a physically tiny amount of each trace mineral, each serves a vital function. Iron helps move oxygen through the blood, zinc is important for blood clotting, and most of the others help chemical processes happen more efficiently.

- chromium
- copper
- fluoride
- iodine
- iron
- manganese
- molybdenum
- selenium
- zinc

PART 2

The Ketogenic Diet

Part 2 will be a basic overview of what the ketogenic diet is and how it affects the human body. We will also look at some of the potentially unpleasant symptoms that people can experience when transitioning from a carbohydrate-heavy diet. While there are ways to mitigate these growing pains, some unaccustomed feelings will be inevitable when switching metabolic energy sources. This section can also be used as a quick-start guide if you want to begin the ketogenic transition before finishing this book.

CHAPTER 4

Mechanics of the Ketogenic Diet

Boiled down to its most basic level, the ketogenic diet is very simple—eat fewer than 50 grams of carbohydrates daily, eat 1.2 to 1.5 grams of protein per kilogram of body weight, and fill in the rest with fat. If you do that, after a few days your body will start relying on fat oxidation and ketone bodies for fuel. Of course, as with all things nutrition, the nuts and bolts are a little more complicated than that. For optimal health, there are considerations other than macronutrient composition.

Because of the late Dr. Robert Atkins and his "diet revolution" that was originally popularized in the early to mid-1970s, the ketogenic diet often comes to mind as the type of short-term diet used for weight-loss purposes. Although this is not what Dr. Atkins intended or advocated for, it is still the net result of his promotion of the ketogenic diet. While a keto-genic diet will almost certainly result in weight loss relatively quickly, it has the potential to be much more than a means to a temporary weight-loss end. I say temporary because if you use the ketogenic diet for weight loss but immediately return to a high-carbohydrate diet, you will most likely gain back any weight you lost as your body again has to deal with the excessive amount of glucose it receives.

The benefits of a ketogenic diet extend beyond weight loss. For example, the medical community has used the ketogenic diet to effectively control epilepsy since the 1920s, when the diet was developed as an alternative to fasting. There are several theories regarding how the ketogenic diet is able to prevent epileptic seizures but there is not currently a consensus. Most likely it has to do with the brain's fuel shift from glucose to fatty acids and ketones.

Recently there has been an explosion of interest in the ketogenic diet's potential uses beyond weight loss and the control of medicinally intractable epilepsy. The ketogenic diet looks to have promising applications for the treatment of a variety of neurological disorders including amyotrophic lateral sclerosis (ALS), multiple sclerosis (MS), Alzheimer's disease, dementia, Parkinson's disease, chronic migraines, and even stroke recovery. It makes perfect sense that the ketogenic diet could provide relief for individuals with these conditions because one of the primary effects of ketosis is a shift in neurologic fuel source, as the common thread between many neurological disorders is some form of glucose metabolism malfunction.

WHAT IS THE KETOGENIC DIET?

The ketogenic diet is awesome.

OK, more in depth: The ketogenic diet is a dietary pattern that shifts your metabolism from relying on glucose as its primary fuel source to relying on fat. This shift is likely an evolutionary trick that humans developed to account for periods in which quick energy was not available and we needed to rely on fat storage to prevent starvation. Almost all of the cells in the body can oxidize, or break down, fat and utilize ketone bodies for fuel instead of the typically preferred glucose. The few cells that do require glucose, including red blood cells (RBC) and certain portions of the brain, can have their needs met by the conversion of protein to glucose.

Even in very lean individuals, the body has a greater capacity to store fat than carbohydrates. The adaptation to burn fat as fuel would have allowed our ancestors to survive the periods in which food was harder to come by.

Typically, your body can store about 2,000 calories of carbohydrate at any given time. Those calories are then converted and stored as about 400 grams of glycogen, which is the stored form of glucose, in skeletal muscle. Muscle glycogen cannot be used by other parts of the body; 100 grams of glycogen stored in the liver can be distributed throughout the body; and 25 grams of glucose circulate in the bloodstream. By contrast, energy stored as fat can easily exceed 10,000 calories, even in lean individuals, and would obviously be of much greater use in those with excess body fat.

Simple arithmetic shows us why a body utilizing fat for its fuel source would be able to keep going much longer than one relying on glucose and glycogen stores. It is for this long-term fuel adaptation that more and more endurance athletes, like ultra-marathon runners and long-distance cyclists, are turning to the ketogenic diet to give them a competitive edge over those that rely on carbohydrate metabolism and must refuel several times during a race.

WHAT DOES THE KETOGENIC DIET DO TO THE BODY?

The ketogenic diet has many physiological effects of great importance. The most obvious effect of the ketogenic diet is in its name—it initiates the production of ketones. Ketones, or ketone bodies, are molecules that are produced during the breakdown of fat that can be used for energy. This metabolic shift has consequences on almost every system in the body. I know you don't want me to detail each one and I'm not going to, but some systems have an important influence on how you will feel while eating the Ketogenic Mediterranean Diet. Let's talk about those.

ENERGY METABOLISM

The primary aspect of a ketogenic diet is that it forces your body to switch from using carbohydrates as its primary source of fuel to using fats instead. This is a two-stage adaptation process and can be a bit of a shock to the system.

First, as you deprive your body of carbohydrates, it will mobilize and disassemble the glycogen stores in your liver to provide glucose to cells throughout the body. The glycogen in your muscles will also get broken down, but it cannot leave the muscles. Once your glycogen stores are depleted, your body will believe itself to be starving and start to break down lean muscle mass so that it can continue to produce glucose. This is why it is recommended that you consume slightly more protein when embarking on a ketogenic diet pattern. Adequate sodium is important for lean mass retention, as well. I'll explain why when discussing electrolyte balance (page 46).

The body cannot break down enough of its lean mass into glucose to cover all of its energy needs, so fatty acid oxidation will increase to make up the deficit. This process of glycogen depletion and fatty acid oxidation initiation will typically take two to three days. You may feel hungry, spaced out, or a bit cranky during this time. Thankfully, this period is brief.

Ketones are a byproduct of fat metabolism. There are certain parts of the body that require glucose. When there is not enough glucose available, the liver can turn protein into glucose to meet these needs. However, the liver itself requires energy in order to make glucose from protein. The liver can break down fat for energy but there are parts of the fat molecule that do not get used. These unused portions are transformed into ketones, which can be used for energy by most of the body's cells.

The second stage of energy metabolism shift is colloquially referred to as fat adaptation, and it usually takes one to three weeks. During this time, the mitochondria in most of the cells of your body are adapting to use fat for energy more efficiently. If you have stayed in uninterrupted ketosis for three weeks, you will likely notice that you no longer get hungry in the same way that you did previously. You will still be hungry, but it will not be as drastic of a transition from high-energy satiety to low-energy hunger. In short, there will be no more carb crashes and no more episodes of feeling "hangry." This is because, as we talked about in the last section, your body has hundreds of thousands of calories stored as fat at any given time. If you are fat adapted, these stores are much easier to access than a constant stream of glucose that needs to be replenished every few hours.

WEIGHT LOSS

As your body transitions from carbohydrate reliance to fatty acid metabolism, you will lose weight. Initially some of this weight will be water weight, because carbohydrates promote water retention and ketosis does the opposite. Beyond that water loss, you will lose some of your fat stores before reaching a stable equilibrium. If weight loss is one of your goals, you will need to eat fewer calories than you burn, just as with a traditional weight-loss plan. However, individuals typically find that adhering to a caloric restriction is easier when following a ketogenic diet pattern because fat leads to greater and longer-lasting feelings of fullness.

There are those who believe that being in ketosis will actually lead to a greater metabolic rate: you will actually burn more calories at rest than when you are eating a carbohydrate-based diet. There may be some truth to the idea that being in ketosis leads to greater weight loss because you are burning more calories, but a more likely explanation is that it is easier to lose weight when following the ketogenic diet because it is easier to adhere to a caloric restriction when eating foods higher in delicious fat. My personal experience with weight loss while eating a ketogenic diet reinforced this theory: When following a caloric restriction plan for the first few months, I was eating about a thousand calories less than the amount needed to maintain weight and I lost roughly two pounds per week during that period. It was delicious and effortless.

In addition to losing weight overall, you can rest assured that the weight you will be losing on a well-formulated ketogenic diet will be primarily fat and not lean mass. There are also indications that, to a greater extent than on a calorically restricted low-fat diet, the fat mass lost during ketosis comes from the abdominal trunk area. Excessive fat stores around the abdomen have been repeatedly associated with the greatest mortality and morbidity risks. Abdominal fat loss is a particularly interesting bit of ketogenic magic because it is the traditional belief that there is no way to target fat loss in a particular region of the body.

BLOOD GLUCOSE AND ENERGY LEVEL REGULATION

Individual reports and well-controlled research show that a ketogenic diet allows for much better blood glucose regulation than does the traditional high-carbohydrate diet pattern. From a physiological perspective, this makes perfect sense. Let's go through it: when you eat carbohydrates they are broken down into glucose, in some cases very quickly, and enter your bloodstream. Your body deals with this glucose in one of four ways:

1. **Burn it**—Glucose can be burned, or metabolized, to be used for immediate energy. Obviously, the amount that your body will burn for immediate energy depends on your energy needs at the time.

2. **Short-term storage**—Glucose can be converted to glycogen and stored in the liver and in the muscles. As mentioned before, these are limited storage solutions, as the muscles collectively can hold about 400 grams of glycogen and the liver taps out at about 100 grams.

3. **Long-term storage**—When your immediate needs are met and your liver and muscle glycogen stores are full, your body will convert carbohydrates into a type of fat tissue

called adipose for indefinite storage. Adipose tissue is what we typically think of as "body fat." If there is an upper limit on the production of adipose tissue, it appears to be so high as to be meaningless.

4. **Get rid of it**—Colloquially referred to as "peeing it out" by my biochemistry professor in college, this is the body's last option for dealing with the excessive glucose loads often thrust upon it by a carbohydrate-heavy diet. Typically, very little glucose leaves the body as waste because the body really likes to store energy, if it can. For most of human history, our food supply was not all that stable and it was not uncommon to rely on stored energy. However, in people that are not producing insulin or have insulin resistance, the body will produce more urine and shed more glucose in order to prevent blood glucose levels from getting dangerously high.

When consuming the SAD, your body is likely making frequent decisions about what to do with more carbohydrates than it can immediately use. The net result of this is often the production of new fat molecules from carbohydrates, called de novo lipogenesis (DNL), and fat storage. The problem is that all four of the above options for handling excess sugars can take several hours. In the time that it takes for these complex and multifaceted chemical processes to take place, you may experience a rise in blood sugar, which can induce negative results.

One to two hours after you eat, your body will have mostly broken down any carbohydrate in your foods and the resulting sugars will have entered your bloodstream. If you ate a lot of carbohydrates, a lot of glucose will enter your bloodstream and need to be dealt with. Some bodies deal with these glycemic loads more efficiently than others, but everyone on a SAD diet experiences at least a short period of time during which blood glucose levels rise before lowering again. Sometimes referred to as the "carb roller-coaster," you may feel highly energetic after a carbohydrate-heavy meal and then very sluggish as your body manages to lower your blood glucose level again.

By contrast, when eating a very-low-carbohydrate ketogenic diet, your body uses the small amount of carbohydrates for brain and RBC fuel, and then makes the rest from protein or the glycerol backbone of triglycerides. This shift from a reactionary regulation of blood glucose levels to a proactive regulation is important. It allows for the body to keep blood glucose levels more even throughout the day, rely less on large loads of insulin, and keeps energy levels more consistent.

ELECTROLYTE REGULATION

Individuals initiating a ketogenic diet often notice that they need to urinate more frequently. Carbohydrates promote water retention, and so carbohydrate restriction and the subsequent breakdown of glycogen, which is anywhere from two-thirds to three-fourths water, results in the production of more urine and the loss of the electrolytes sodium, potassium, and magnesium. Additionally, insulin levels play a role in controlling how much sodium is retained. Lower insulin levels lead to a greater excretion of sodium by the kidneys.

Here is where the connection between sodium and lean muscle mass preservation comes in. Your body uses two types of cations, which are positively charged ions, to regulate the pressure and fluid levels between the fluid inside your cells (intracellular fluid) and the fluid outside of cells (extracellular fluid). These two cations are sodium and potassium.

Sodium is the dominant cation in the extracellular fluid, and potassium is the dominant cation in the intracellular fluid. In order for your blood pressure to stay high enough and for your muscles to work properly, the balance of sodium and potassium has to be constant.

When your kidneys begin to excrete more sodium due to the physiological changes of ketosis, this balance can be thrown off. In an attempt to preserve this balance, the body will begin to excrete potassium, as well. The problem is that in order to do this, it needs to break down lean tissue to free the potassium. Therefore, if you do not properly replenish sodium while in ketosis, you run the risk of muscle loss driven by the body's need for electrolyte balance.

Sodium, potassium, and magnesium are critically important to a whole host of functions within the body and their concentrations within the body are equally important. Too much or too little can be problematic, and mild deficiency of one or all three can cause some of the negative side effects associated with the initiation phase of ketosis. Often referred to as the "keto flu," these side effects can involve low energy, headaches, muscle cramps, rapid heartbeat, constipation, and diarrhea. All of these symptoms can be explained by an electrolyte imbalance. In fact, the keto flu can be avoided altogether with electrolyte supplementation and replenishment. In *The Art and Science of Low Carbohydrate Living*, the authors recommend consuming five grams of sodium per day and taking a slow-release magnesium supplement.

Potassium should not be an issue for you while eating the Ketogenic Mediterranean Diet because you should be able to get adequate potassium from the copious amount of delicious vegetables you'll consume.

BLOOD LIPID REGULATION

Blood lipids include triglyceride and cholesterol levels. Triglycerides are a type of fat that your body uses for long-term storage. They are called triglycerides because they have a glycerol backbone with three fatty acids attached, causing them to look like an uppercase E. High triglyceride levels in the blood after an overnight fast are strongly associated with increased cardiovascular disease risk. The main factor in the elevation of fasting serum triglycerides is carbohydrate consumption. Carbohydrate restriction and ketosis have been shown to lower triglyceride blood levels very effectively. If you think about it, this makes perfect sense; when your body is relying on fat for fuel, there will be less available to hang out in your bloodstream.

Traditionally we think of cholesterol in three ways: total cholesterol, low-density lipoprotein cholesterol (LDL-C), and high-density lipoprotein cholesterol (HDL-C).

TOTAL CHOLESTEROL. This is the combined HDL-C and LDL-C circulating in your blood at any given time. Unfortunately, this number is not very useful for risk prediction. Generally speaking, clinicians will tell you that you should aim for your total cholesterol number to be equal to or less than two hundred milligrams of cholesterol per deciliter of blood. However, without more information, this number really doesn't tell us anything about cardiovascular risk.

LDL-C. Both LDL-C and HDL-C are actually fats and proteins combined—that's why they are called lipoproteins. Anyway, LDL-C is thought of as the "bad" type of cholesterol that you want to minimize and is associated with a greater risk of cardiovascular disease. It is thought that the reason higher LDL-C blood levels are associated with higher cardiovascular risk is that LDL-C can build up on arterial walls and restrict blood flow over time.

HDL-C. High-density lipoprotein is thought to be the "good" variety of cholesterol and higher numbers are associated with lower risk. We believe HDL-C to be "good" because it travels through the bloodstream collecting cholesterol and transports it out of the bloodstream.

Importantly, the ratio of total cholesterol to HDL-C seems to be a better predictor of risk than any of these numbers alone. The ideal ratio is said to be less than 3.5 to 1.

Emerging science in the area of cholesterol and heart disease tells us that this picture is much more nuanced than we currently understand. As with most advances in knowledge, research findings take a long time to make it into common practice but our understanding of the complex role of fats in our diets is getting better all the time. One thing that research has consistently shown is that the ketogenic diet reduces serum triglyceride levels, decreases LDL-C, and increases HDL-C.

APO A AND APO B. I mentioned above that HDL-C and LDL-C are actually combinations of fat and proteins. Apolipoprotein A (apo A) is a constituent found in HDL-C, and apolipoprotein B (apo B) is found in LDL-C. Researchers have been finding that the ratio of apo B to apo A is a better predictor of cardiovascular risk than that of HDL-C to total cholesterol. However, reference ranges have not been standardized and testing is still not widely used. Ask your physician about this test and ratio if you are curious. This will both spread awareness of its use, if your physician is not yet aware, and increase your knowledge of your particular cardiovascular risk.

LDL-P. While LDL-C measures the concentration of cholesterol in the particles of LDL, it does nothing to indicate the actual number of LDL particles. That's what the P in LDL-P is: particles. This is a measurement of how many LDL particles are in your blood. Interestingly, this looks to be an even more accurate predictor of cardiovascular risk than any of the previously mentioned ratios. Early evidence indicates that the ketogenic diet improves LDL-P levels, as well. However, research still needs to be done before any type of clinical usefulness can arise from this measure.

CHAPTER 5

What to Eat

When I ramble on about the physiology and metabolic mechanisms behind the changes most of us will feel when embarking upon a ketogenic diet pattern, eventually everyone interrupts me with this question: but what do you actually eat?!

That's a fair question. A ketogenic diet is very difficult for a lot of people to wrap their minds around since they have been told for most (if not all) of their lives that dietary fat will kill them and should be avoided.

For those looking for a quick start with the ketogenic diet, let's briefly talk about what will and will not fit into a ketogenic diet plan. Later, we'll discuss these topics in more detail.

FOODS THAT DO NOT FIT A KETOGENIC DIET PLAN

It is easiest to start with the foods that have no place in a ketogenic diet. Here is a quick list of things to be omitted:

- grains
- legumes
- most fruits
- starchy vegetables
- sugars

Let's break that down a bit. If you can't eat any sugars, grains, starchy vegetables, legumes, and most fruits, you also can't eat many of the following:

- baked goods
- beans
- breads
- candies
- cow's and goat's milk
- pastas
- potatoes

I realize that upon reading that list, many of you had the urge to throw this book across the room. I accept that and hope we can move past it.

The ketogenic diet and any diet based on it, like the Ketogenic Mediterranean Diet, *must* be a very-low-carbohydrate diet. There is no way around it. Carbohydrates suppress ketone production. As one who has been eating the ketogenic diet for over a year, believe me, I understand how daunting it sounds to give up all of the sweets and sweetened things in our modern diet. Also believe me when I say it is worth it.

FOODS THAT WILL FIT A KETOGENIC DIET PLAN

The foods that will make up the majority of your diet include non-starchy vegetables, fatty fruits and their oils, nuts and seeds, eggs, dairy excluding milk, fish, and other meats. Non-starchy vegetables include just about all vegetables except potatoes, sweet potatoes, carrots, and corn. Fatty fruits would be avocados, coconuts, and olives. Berries may be included in moderation. Nuts and seeds will be useful but must also be eaten in moderation, as they have a moderate amount of carbohydrate content, depending on the variety. Almost all cheeses and some yogurts can fit nicely within a ketogenic diet plan. Look for Greek yogurt and make sure it is not sweetened, because many commercial yogurt varieties have outrageous amounts of sugar added.

Don't make assumptions about a food product's carbohydrate content if you are dealing with anything that has a label. The nature of the industrialized food supply in the United States is, to use a technical term, nutzo. Sugars or corn derivatives are added to just about everything. Here are some examples of processed foods that have more carbohydrates than they rightfully should because of added sweeteners.

- ▶ beef jerky
- ▶ dressings
- ▶ ketchup
- ▶ peanut butter

- ▶ processed cheeses
- ▶ sausages
- ▶ tomato sauce
- ▶ yogurt

Using the broad strokes painted above, put together meals such that you do not exceed twenty grams of net carbohydrate daily for at least three weeks, at which time you may be able to increase your daily amount to as much as fifty grams. Your particular carbohydrate tolerance is unique, but for this diet I recommend that it fall within the range of twenty to fifty grams per day.

Net carbohydrate is the term used for the amount of carbohydrate that the body can actually digest. Because we cannot digest fiber, we do not have to count the fiber portion of the carbohydrates we eat toward our daily total. To determine net carbohydrate, subtract the grams of fiber from the total carbohydrates. This method is not universally accepted within the ketogenic community because of variability between how different bodies metabolize fiber. I recommend using the net carbohydrate method, but you should try to give yourself three to five grams of wiggle room per day. See Chapter 10 for specific recipes and Chapter 11 for a meal plan.

Strangely enough, there are a couple of almost-carbohydrates that can fit within a ketogenic diet plan for some people. Sugar alcohols and non-nutritive sweeteners can be useful additions to a ketogenic diet plan because they can be utilized in desserts and drinks if you occasionally crave something sweet. However, as you will read, they should be used sparingly and you will need to experiment with them to find your level of tolerance.

SUGAR ALCOHOLS

Sugar alcohols are not sugars at all, but polyols that occur naturally or are derived from sugars through chemical processes. They are used as sweeteners or thickeners and tend to be less sweet than table sugar. The body does not metabolize sugar alcohols very well, but they will provide some calories when eaten. Though they are generally regarded as diabetic and keto safe, they do raise blood glucose levels and inhibit ketone production in some individuals. They also commonly cause bloating or diarrhea if you consume too much. Unfortunately I can't tell you what "too much" means, because they tend to affect people differently. You'll just have to experiment and see how you react. You can spot them on labels because they all end with –ol. Some commonly used sugar alcohols are erythritol, glycerol, mannitol, and xylitol.

NON-NUTRITIVE SWEETENERS. These appear in almost anything with the word "diet" on it. They are called non-nutritive because, like sugar alcohols, the body does not completely metabolize them and they don't provide much in the way of nutrition. None of the non-nutritive sweeteners raise blood glucose levels or interfere with ketone production.

The use and ingestion of non-nutritive sweeteners is a topic that people tend to feel very passionately about. Over the years, there have been anecdotal accounts of these substances being linked with everything from migraines to obesity to cancer. The problem is, there is no quality clinical evidence to back these claims up. I believe that it is best to avoid these in favor of developing a palate that is less accustomed to sweetness, but I do not think that occasionally consuming them will do you any harm. The FDA has approved the use of these sweeteners:

- acesulfame-K (Sweet One)
- aspartame (NutraSweet and Equal)
- neotame
- saccharin (Sweet'N Low)
- sucralose (Splenda)
- stevia (Truvia and PureVia)

WHAT A KETOGENIC DIET IS NOT

There are a few things that you will undoubtedly encounter repeatedly once you embark on a ketogenic diet pattern. I do not know why these myths surrounding ketogenic diets are so pervasive, but I suspect it has something to do with how different the ketogenic diet is from what people have been told all their lives. Regardless, I want to take a moment to make very clear what the ketogenic diet is *not*.

KETOACIDOSIS. Typically, this is the first point of confusion that needs to be clarified for friends and family. Ketoacidosis is a potentially deadly condition that insulin-dependent diabetics (type I and advanced type II) are at risk of developing if they do not get enough exogenous insulin. Basically, glucose cannot travel from the bloodstream and into the cells that need it, so the body begins to make ketones as it does when actually deprived of carbohydrates. Danger occurs because insulin is also the hormone used to stop ketone production. In the absence of insulin, ketone production can run unchecked and eventually reach a point in which the pH of the blood is affected by the excessive amount of ketone bodies present. Because ketone bodies are slightly acidic, their accumulation will drive the pH of the blood down, which can very quickly result in coma or death.

In individuals that have functioning insulin-producing and storing beta cells on their pancreas, ketoacidosis will not occur. To borrow an example from Dr. Peter Attia, a medical doctor studying diet and longevity, nutritional ketosis and ketoacidosis are similar in the way that a nice toasty fire in a fireplace and an uncontrolled house fire are similar. They are both fire and both provide heat energy, but one is safe, beneficial, and contained, while the other is out of control and potentially deadly.

A STEAK AND BACON DIET. Honestly, of all of the misconceptions about a ketogenic diet, this one bothers me the most. As a former vegan who understands the inescapably negative environmental consequences of our nation's current level of meat consumption, it makes me want to Hulk-smash when I hear a morning talk show host describe the ketogenic diet as an "all bacon" or "steak and bacon" diet. You could technically only eat steak and bacon and you would certainly be in ketosis. However, your proportion of saturated fat to monounsaturated fat intake would not be optimized for longevity, you would likely be missing several important micronutrients, your food bill would skyrocket, you would be disproportionately contributing to global warming, and you'd get really bored.

A HIGH-PROTEIN DIET. While it is true that you need to eat more protein than the standard daily recommended 0.8 grams per kilogram of body weight (in ketosis, you would probably increase your protein consumption to something closer to 1.2 to 1.5 grams per kilogram), it is by no means a high-protein diet. The ratios of your macronutrients should fall somewhere around 70 percent fat, 10 to 20 percent protein, and 5 to 10 percent carbohydrate. This should be described as a high-fat, moderate-protein, very-low-carbohydrate diet.

WHY USE THE KETOGENIC DIET?

A well-formulated ketogenic diet is an amazing metabolic tool that will lead to changes in the way you look and feel. More than that, it produces very real physiological changes that have incredible implications for weight management, heart and brain health, and longevity. Unfortunately, it is also almost completely opposite to the dietary and health advice that our government has been selling for the past 45 years. This can produce quite a lot of cognitive dissonance in the discerning eater.

I whole-heartedly believe that for many people, a ketogenic diet (particularly the Ketogenic Mediterranean Diet) is the healthiest possible way to eat. Even with my education, clinical experience, and this belief, I still have moments when I think, "Goodness, I'm eating too much fat!" Don't worry; if you were raised in the United States, these moments are natural. Fat has been the enemy all our lives. But this fervor for low-fat everything was more politically motivated than it was scientifically based. The evidence behind anti-fat rhetoric is sorely lacking, and the American people have been the subjects of a vast dietary experiment.

Unlike any other dietary pattern, the ketogenic diet is an all-or-nothing endeavor. Strictly speaking, you are free to have "cheat days" where you eat enough carbohydrates for your body to stop ketosis, but if you choose to do so you will most likely need to go through the initiation and adaptation phases again. That hardly seems worth it for a slice of pizza. This fact can be a bit off-putting to some people but as you will see in the coming chapters, once you start living the high-fat, high-energy, and fantastically delicious Ketogenic Mediterranean Diet, you will have no desire to go back to the Standard American Diet and the energy roller-coaster, excess weight, and increased risk of disease that come with it.

A ketogenic diet is not for everyone because not all of us have issues with the metabolism of carbohydrates. However, I think there is a good argument to be made that somewhere in the range of two thirds of the population does not deal with excessive carbohydrate intake very well. If you are one of these individuals, a ketogenic diet is the way to take back control of your health.

PART 3

The Mediterranean Diet

The Mediterranean diet does not drastically alter your metabolism the way that the ketogenic diet does. There is no fuel source change, no increase in fatty acid metabolism, and no subsequent increase in electrolyte loss. With this in mind, there will be much less discussion of biology and chemical processes in this section.

CHAPTER 6

Food and History

The Mediterranean diet is an eating pattern replete with copious amounts of various fruits and vegetables, whole grains, nuts and seeds, seafood, and certain types of fats. It also contains moderate amounts of lean meats, dairy, and alcohol. Usually it contains very little processed food, particularly processed grains and sweeteners, and proportionally less red meat than does the SAD. Most of the foods included are whole and fresh, and spices are used much more liberally than salt. Here are some examples of foods regularly eaten by those following a Mediterranean diet:

- almonds
- avocado
- barley
- beans
- berries
- couscous
- eggs
- herring
- oats
- olives
- pork
- poultry
- salmon
- tofu
- trout

Obviously, some of the foods mentioned above are not compatible with the ketogenic diet because they are too carbohydrate heavy. This includes all of the grains, because even 100 percent whole grains are metabolized into glucose and will inhibit ketone production. The majority of the fruits in the Mediterranean diet must also be excluded due to their sugar content. This is not to say that these foods cannot be part of a healthful eating pattern, just not one that utilizes ketosis. I will still be discussing these elements of the diet in this chapter because they are an integral part of the traditional Mediterranean diet. Just keep in mind that as we move on to the Ketogenic Mediterranean Diet, we'll be making some changes.

Although there is none of the metabolic wizardry associated with a ketogenic diet, the Mediterranean diet is also a very healthful diet. It is associated with lower body weight, decreased risk of metabolic and cardiovascular diseases, and lower all-cause mortality. This section will explore the history and promotion of the Mediterranean diet and associated lifestyle, what health benefits are associated with this lifestyle, and what the likely explanations for these benefits are.

It is common practice for media outlets to claim amazing benefits from small dietary changes, sometimes with just a single food item, or even just a single nutrient! Unfortunately, life and health are more complicated than that. To realize actual, sustainable changes in health and well-being, we must make *behavioral* changes to reflect our goals.

Many diets are healthful and delicious on their own, but to experience optimal health, some general lifestyle changes are required. In fact, the name "Mediterranean diet" is a bit misleading, since many of the physical and mental benefits associated with it require lifestyle adjustments modeled after the habits of the diet's originators. For this reason, I will also be discussing the associated physical activity and mindfulness practices that are a part of Mediterranean lifestyle.

HISTORY

It is nearly impossible to pin down a date that the Mediterranean diet was created because it is the result of years and years of cultural heritage passed from generation to generation. Adding to the difficulty, "Mediterranean" refers to a region, not one unified culture. It could be argued that any of the dozens of countries on the Mediterranean Sea, including Algeria, Israel, and Turkey, practice Mediterranean diets. The list of countries that have existed in this region over the thousands of years of human civilization is even more overwhelming. Thankfully, for the sake of both of our sanity, it is much easier to trace *when* the diet and lifestyle called Mediterranean was originally promoted than *where*.

Though the diet was originally developed in the 1960s and based upon the typical eating patterns found in Greece, Southern Italy, and Spain in the 1940s, it was not widely promoted until Ancel Keys studied it in 1975 and did not gain much traction until the 1990s. Keys was the most aggressive proponent of the idea that dietary fat and cholesterol are responsible for heart disease, which is somewhat ironic because the Mediterranean diet as we know it today actually contains more fat calories than the low-fat dogma recommends.

Keys was a heavy promoter of this diet because of his interpretation of the "Seven Countries Study," which he directed. The data from this observational study appeared to show that the inhabitants of the island of Crete had significantly lower incidence of heart disease than Americans. Though many (including myself) now believe Keys made mistakes in his analysis of the data, we are lucky that Keys picked up the Mediterranean diet because the attention that he drew to the diet is likely the only reason we are aware of it now.

Though Keys' efforts to promote the Mediterranean diet were not terribly effective at the time, he did draw enough attention to it for the public health community to be aware. One of the thought leaders of this community, Dr. Walter Willett of the Harvard School of Public Health, began promoting the diet again in the 1990s. This time, the public was much more receptive to this diet rich in whole foods, olive oil, and fish. In 1993, the Harvard School of Public Health teamed up with the food and nutrition educational nonprofit Oldways to standardize what we now think of as the Mediterranean diet. Oldways developed and released the Mediterranean Diet Pyramid at this time, as well.

Physical activity and a sense of community are included as the base of the lifestyle. The largest portion of the diet itself is made of vegetables, fruits, nuts and seeds, olive oil, and whole grains. Then, moving toward the smaller tip of the pyramid, you have fish and seafood products; poultry, eggs, and dairy live in the next section; and finally, at the top, you'll find red meat and sweets of all kinds. Located outside the pyramid are wine and water as beverages.

There was initially a good deal of skepticism regarding the acceptance of this diet pattern because high-quality olive oil, hummus, tabbouleh, and various whole grains were not widely used or all that easy to purchase in the early nineties. Despite this doubt, the Mediterranean diet has only grown in popularity. Because Harvard and Oldways, the main promoters of the diet, were incredibly well respected, health professionals fell in love with this diet and began to recommend it to their patients. Of course, the hundreds of published studies touting the health benefits helped quite a bit, as well.

As the popularity of the Mediterranean diet grew, the market responded and products associated with it became more accessible. Depending on your age and how much attention you pay to the grocery aisles, you may have noticed that things like olive oils and marinated oils, sun-dried tomatoes, hummus, a greater variety of grains, and other novel items have become ubiquitous. Greek yogurt is a good example. Greek yogurt was so obscure in the early nineties that I could not even find market data for it at that time. The first company to market its yogurt as Greek was Fage in 1998, just five years after the introduction of the Mediterranean diet pyramid. Since then, the market has grown steadily. Sales of Greek yogurt alone are expected to reach four billion by 2019. I'm not saying the Mediterranean diet's popularity is directly responsible for the increase in Greek yogurt's share of the market, but it is a good metric that indicates a rise in interest in Mediterranean diet-associated foods.

CHAPTER 7

Lifestyle Aspects

The food of the Mediterranean diet is but a small portion of what makes it unique. There are many important lifestyle factors associated with the diet that likely play just as important a role in the health and wellness benefits of the diet as the food itself. The combined effect of these habits appears to be a lowered risk of heart disease and all-cause mortality, a lower average body mass index, and, more subjectively, reduced stress levels and a greater sense of life satisfaction.

The main lifestyle factors that are important to a Mediterranean diet lifestyle are physical activity, abstention from tobacco use, low to moderate alcohol usage, longer meal times, and a strong sense of community. I'm sure living close to beautiful beaches doesn't hurt, either. Beach proximity aside, we will be carrying these factors over to the Ketogenic Mediterranean lifestyle, so let's use this opportunity to get better acquainted with each one.

PHYSICAL ACTIVITY. Walking, leisure sports, and manual labor around the house are common aspects of life in many parts of the Mediterranean, and, subsequently, residents of that region do not struggle to meet the recommended daily amount of physical activity. Exercise can certainly be about performance and pushing your limits, but for our purposes it is more about baseline wellness. You can pick any metric, from mental well-being to lung capacity to bone strength, and it will be positively correlated with regular physical activity. Of course, correlation is not good enough. In this case, however, there are many well-described physiological mechanisms responsible for these benefits. I will offer some prescriptions for ways to incorporate more physical activity into your daily routine in the next section and point you to some great resources if you are interested in understanding these mechanisms.

TOBACCO USE. In this day and age, there are very few people left that deny the many negative health consequences of tobacco product usage. In spite of this apparent understanding, the use of tobacco products is still more widespread than it should be in the United States. If you are a smoker or use smokeless tobacco products (like chewing tobacco, known as dip), cessation of these products is the single best lifestyle change that you can make to reduce your risk of early death or debility. The recent rise in using e-cigarettes as a smoking alternative, or "vaping," certainly seems like an improvement, but early research indicates that it does not come without risks of its own. Total cessation is the best policy.

MODERATE ALCOHOL USE. Moderate alcohol use means no more than one to two servings daily, and in the traditional Mediterranean diet, alcohol means red wine. This is likely a good example of correlation but not causation. There is no evidence that I am aware of indicating that there is anything uniquely beneficial to red wine itself. While it is included in traditional Mediterranean diets and traditional Mediterranean diets seem to be protective against a whole host of negative health outcomes, it has only been assumed that red wine is in some way protective. It has been theorized that the antioxidant content of the flavonoids in the skins of the grapes may be a factor. My theory is that a good glass of red wine is divine and when it is enjoyed with friends or family, it is even better. The improved mood and life quality experienced while enjoying that glass of wine likely lowers stress levels, which in turn lowers inflammation. Lowered inflammation is absolutely protective against disease.

Regardless of the mechanisms at play, if you enjoy red wine you should feel free to continue enjoying it while pursuing a Mediterranean diet. However, this is one of those situations in which you can have too much of a good thing. One to two glasses is associated with good health, but any more than that results in diminishing returns. Additionally, one five-ounce serving of red wine contains four grams of carbohydrates, so you'll want to enjoy it in moderation for sure.

LONGER MEAL TIMES. People enjoying the Mediterranean lifestyle do a better job of remembering that meals are not only a time to nourish the body, but can also be a fantastic way to take a brief repose from the stress of the day and nourish the mind. Because it takes at least 20 minutes for your brain to register the chemical signals your body manufactures to indicate that you are full, enjoying your meals more slowly also allows for better portion control. If you slow down while eating, you give yourself time to relish your meal and listen to the cues from your body that tell you when you're full. This ties into the concept of "mindful eating," which I will discuss in greater detail in the next section. For now, we'll just say there is no place in the Mediterranean diet for standing in front of your fridge stuffing cold falafel in your mouth before running off to do errands.

COMMUNITY. It is difficult to overstate the incredible and far-reaching effects that a strong sense of community can have on your health. Multiple studies have noted a correlation between having a place in a community and having higher life satisfaction scores, increased happiness ratings, and more positive health outcomes.

Maslow's hierarchy of needs, the famous theory of human motivation, organizes human needs into a pyramid with physiological needs like food and water at the bottom and the idea of "self-actualization," or the realization of one's talents, at the top. But just below this need to use our talents is the need for esteem, or a sense of belonging. In other words, we think of a sense of community as a basic human need. That goes a long way toward explaining why the strong sense of community associated with the Mediterranean lifestyle would lower stress and be correlated with better health.

We will focus on this aspect in the following section. In a society that has been told for the last 40 years that fat is bad, eating a diet that is 70 to 80 percent fat can be understandably isolating. Thankfully, there are ways to mitigate this isolation by finding a community and enjoying the wonderful feeling of sharing a meal with loved ones.

THE MEDITERRANEAN DIET IS SO MUCH MORE

The Mediterranean diet as we know it was manufactured by the Harvard School of Public Health and Oldways, the food and nutritional education organization. It represents an intentional effort on the part of the public health community to take their observations of populations that tend to be very healthy and make them accessible to a broader audience. Thankfully, the subsequent popularity of the diet has prompted food manufacturers and importers to widen the variety of foods that are readily available, making it easier than ever to follow a Mediterranean diet.

While the eating pattern has been the most heavily studied aspect of this lifestyle, I still feel that it is inappropriate to refer to it only as a "diet" because of the lifestyle aspects that are a necessary component. Thankfully, none of these lifestyle changes are outside our reach. They can all be implemented relatively easily with the right guidance. Regular physical activity, cessation of tobacco use, the inclusion of (or restriction to) a moderate amount of alcohol, more mindful eating, and a sense of community are all beneficial habits regardless of the diet you are pursuing.

It is time to take the Mediterranean lifestyle to the next level and incorporate the principles of the ketogenic diet. Carbohydrate restriction and inclusion of the right kind of fats, combined with the whole-foods and flavor-rich approach of Mediterranean cuisine, will yield amazing health benefits without any sense of sacrifice. It is high time we explore what these two amazing dietary plans can be when combined.

PART 4

The Ketogenic Mediterranean Diet

So far we have discussed the basic nuts and bolts of what food is, what the body does with food once it's ingested, the traditional ketogenic diet with its metabolic changes, and the traditional Mediterranean diet and associated lifestyle. Now it is time to integrate these subjects and combine the best of the ketogenic diet and the best of the Mediterranean diet to make the Ketogenic Mediterranean Diet. In Part 4, you'll learn how to incorporate the diet into your life, a slew of recipes, tips for traveling and eating out, and a seven-day meal plan. I'll also discuss ways to incorporate more physical activity into your daily routine without doing "exercise," strategies for stress management, and ways to share your new eating pattern with friends and family.

CHAPTER 8

What to Eat on the Ketogenic Mediterranean Diet

The Ketogenic Mediterranean Diet is a powerful hybrid of the only dietary approach that actually changes the way your mitochondria process and prioritize fuel and a diet associated with longer life and happier people. It uses the most important parts of the ketogenic diet, carbohydrate restriction and fat inclusion, and the most crucial parts of the Mediterranean diet, whole foods and a whole-life approach, to make a delicious and sustainable way of living and eating. It is the Prius of diets, except it's more fun than a Prius. But it *is* energy efficient. Anyway, you get the idea.

Whole foods are those that have been as minimally pro-cessed as possible. These are easier to include in this diet because they are easier to control. For example, if you start with peanuts, put them in a processor with some oil and salt, and grind them up, you know what is in your peanut butter: peanuts, oil, and salt. If you purchase premade peanut butter, you cannot make the assumption that peanuts, oil, and salt are the only ingredients. Of course, the nutrition label and ingredient list is a great resource for processed foods, but it is not always a perfect system.

Let's say you want some peanut chicken and you, a diligent consumer, look at the ingredients to make sure you are comfortable with everything in this dish. Peanut butter may be one of those ingredients, but the ingredients of the peanut butter itself may not be listed. Did they make that peanut butter with palm oil? Did they use sugar? There is no way to know.

Another point to consider when thinking about whole versus processed foods is that manufacturers are not required to tell you what they did to the ingredients listed. For example, if you purchase ground beef patties from some of the largest US meat producers, those patties may have been sprayed with ammonia as one of the last steps of processing. There is no requirement that you be informed of this fun fact when you are purchasing this type of meat.

But that's enough of the gross reasons to avoid processed foods when you can. Let's just agree that whole foods are, as a whole (you see what I did there?), a better choice for the Ketogenic Mediterranean Diet.

So what should you actually eat? To borrow a simplification from food journalist Michael Pollan: "Eat food. Not too much. Mostly plants." And I'll add: "Lots of fat!" Specifically, you'll want to be eating 70 to 80 percent fat, 10 to 20 percent protein, and 5 to 10 percent carbohydrates. Be sure to note that I stand by the "mostly plants" portion of Michael Pollan's statement, and recall that a ketogenic diet should not be a "mostly meat" diet. Neither your body nor your planet could sustain an all-meat diet.

At the same time, this is not necessarily a vegetarian diet, but it can easily be converted to a vegetarian diet if that is appealing to you. However, if you lean in the full vegan direction and prefer no animal-derived products of any kind…stop reading this book. It is my opinion that a very-low-carbohydrate vegan diet would be unsustainably restrictive and likely lead to nutrient deficiencies. Plus, if you avoided carbohydrates and all animal products, your level of smugness would likely be unbearable.

Your plates should be mostly filled with non-starchy vegetables such as:

- asparagus
- broccoli
- cauliflower
- cucumbers
- kale
- mushrooms
- onions
- spinach and other greens
- tomatoes
- zucchini

The vegetables will often be coated or cooked in some type of delicious fat, like olive or coconut oil, cream or nut-based sauces, or butter or cheese. There should also be fatty fruits like olives and avocados on many of your plates.

You should include protein in every meal. Good protein sources are:

- cheese and dairy, like yogurt
- eggs
- all meats, including poultry and fish
- meat alternatives, like tofu and tempeh
- certain nuts and nut butters

Snacks and garnishes will often come from nuts and seeds like almonds and sunflower seeds. Though you may not believe me until you actually taste some of what is available, there are some amazing possibilities for desserts, as well. You can easily make ice cream, fudge, cakes, cookies, and more once you get a hang of the necessary cooking skillset. As you will see as we get into the specifics, there is almost no end to the variety of foods you will be able to create and enjoy once you get more comfortable with fats.

BUYING FOOD WISELY

Before we begin, it might be helpful to discuss some of the purchasing considerations you'll need to pay attention to when shopping for your Ketogenic Mediterranean Diet. Because our food supply system is, as I said before, nutzo, there are going to be some additional considerations for all of the food you buy. I'll be discussing things to look for and avoid in all the categories of food featured below.

BUYING FRUITS AND VEGETABLES

FRESH PRODUCE. Most fruits and vegetables begin losing nutrient value the minute they are picked, so the best time to get produce is when it's ripe, fresh-picked, and at its prime nutritional value. Then, it should be eaten immediately. If you are buying from a farmers market or community supported agriculture program (CSA), you are likely getting produce that was at best picked a few hours before you bought it and at worst a few days earlier. These are the ideal conditions for produce consumption. Of course, you still need to be sure to rinse your purchases well, because almost every grower uses a pesticide or herbicide of some kind that could leave residue on the leaves or skin of your produce.

If you are buying from a grocery store, the situation is a little different. Many times the produce that you find on supermarket shelves is picked before it is ripe and at its most nutritious because it may need to travel several hundred miles before reaching your local store. After the long truck ride to the store, it can sit on the shelves for a few more days before you pick it up and take it home. Then, at home, it may sit in the fridge for a bit longer before finally being eaten. The type of "fresh" that you find in the supermarket may have lost up to 45 percent of its nutritional value before it gets eaten. Yikes!

FLASH FROZEN FOODS. Alternately, produce that has undergone the process of flash freezing retains much more of its nutritional content. These fruits and vegetables were typically picked when ripe, and then processed and flash frozen immediately. Flash freezing is a process in which the temperature is lowered so quickly that things become frozen in a matter of seconds—or, you could say, in a flash! This quick freezing allows the nutrients that are present at peak ripeness to be "locked in" until the vegetables are thawed.

PRESERVED FOODS. Canning, pickling, and dehydrating are other preservation techniques. Canning is not ideal for vegetables because the vegetables are typically cooked and stored in a brine, which is a very salty liquid. This can rob them of much of their nutritional value, texture, and flavor. Likewise, canned or jarred fruits will often be packed in sugary syrup. Additionally, some cans are lined with chemicals that may leach into your produce as they age in the can. This is typically true of acidic foods like tomatoes.

Pickling is a process that I barely count as preservation because while it does preserve whatever you are pickling well beyond its natural shelf life, the pickling process fundamentally changes the nutrient content, texture, and flavor profile of whatever is being pickled. Instead of thinking of pickling as preservation, just think of it as creating a new version of the produce you've used. Pickled green beans are not very similar to fresh, frozen, or canned green beans. Importantly for us, the pickled version of whatever it is may contain significantly more sugar than the fresh, frozen, or canned varieties.

When shopping for fruits, there is an additional consideration to be aware of: avoid dried varieties. Dehydrating fruit removes the water and concentrates the carbohydrate content. This means that it becomes much easier to accidentally exceed your carbohydrate limit when enjoying dried berries. For example, one ounce of fresh blueberries contains about three net grams of carbohydrate, but one ounce of dried blueberries has a little over 20 net grams.

So, to recap how you should prioritize preservation methods based on nutrient value when shopping for fruits and vegetables:

1. Local and fresh from your garden, local farmers market, or CSA.

2. Flash frozen from a supermarket.

3. Fresh from a supermarket.

4. Canned.

As you can see, pickled and dehydrated are not on the list because we decided they don't count.

I know that for many fruits and vegetables, freezing and thawing will change the texture in less-than-pleasant ways. I get it, frozen food is not appropriate for all applications. You're still doing great if you eat supermarket fresh.

ORGANIC VERSUS CONVENTIONAL. From a nutritional perspective, there is no evidence that there is much of a difference between organic and conventional vegetables. There is, however, some evidence that conventional produce has more residual pesticide on it than organic does. If you wash your vegetables well, chemical residue won't be much of an issue. However, I choose organic whenever possible because the farming practices used in organic farming are much better for the planet, and the types of pesticides and herbicides used are typically less toxic to humans. In my opinion and experience, organic varieties tend to be more flavorful than their conventional counterparts, as well. No matter which you choose, rinse thoroughly.

GENETICALLY MODIFIED ORGANISMS. Genetically modified organisms (GMOs) are organisms that have been altered on the genetic level in order to provide a trait or characteristic that the manipulator desires. This is achieved by taking genes from an organism that has the desired trait and splicing them into the genetic code of another organism. For example, Bt soy and Bt corn are varieties of soy and corn that have had genes added from the bacteria *Bacillus thuringiensis* (commonly referred to as Bt) because this bacteria is naturally toxic to certain pests. Thus, through genetic engineering, Bt soy and Bt corn do not need to have as much pesticide sprayed on them because they produce their own. This is but one example. There are thousands of varieties of GMOs on the market now, and their special traits affect anything from flavor to growing speed to pest resistance.

To date, there is no good evidence that GMOs are in any way dangerous to humans or are less nutritious than their non-GMO counterparts. In fact, genetic modification has been used to make some crops more nutritious. Take golden rice, for example. Golden rice is a variety of genetically modified rice that, through manipulation, contains beta-carotene in its grains. Beta-carotene is the precursor to vitamin A; during digestion, beta-carotene is converted to the essential vitamin. Golden rice is being developed to make vitamin A more easily accessible to the populations that are most affected by vitamin A deficiency.

Of course, if you have seen any news source in the past few years, you know that GMOs are a very controversial issue. Many argue that GMOs cause detrimental health effects, or that we cannot yet know what the long-term effects of consuming them will be. Others, myself included, are concerned about the potential unforeseen consequences that GMOs may have on the ecosystem.

Regardless of which side of the GMO issue you find yourself on, it is currently rather difficult to avoid consuming GMO foods. At the time of this writing, producers in the United States are not required to label whether or not a food contains GMOs. The only way to be sure that the fruits and vegetables you are buying do not contain GMOs is to purchase USDA organic varieties. One of the requirements of this label is that the food item contains no genetically modified components. Another label to look for is the "Non-GMO Project Verified" label. This denotes that the food item has been verified to have less than one percent GMO ingredients.

Because of the prevalence of GMO crops, you are safe to assume that if a food or food product is not labeled organic or Non-GMO Project Verified, it contains GMOs or is a genetically modified organism. However, based on the huge movement for labeling and the current political climate, I imagine that by the time this book is published, GMO labeling will be required in the United States and therefore making an informed choice in the grocery store will be easier.

Nuance and controversy of GMOs aside, the carbohydrate content of GMO and non-GMO foods will not differ, so until such a time that the evidence about the health effects of GMOs is more conclusive, you'll just have to make up your own mind about them.

BUYING PROTEINS

Just as with fruits and vegetables, purchasing proteins from local producers is preferable to shopping exclusively at the supermarket. Local producers are more likely to be able to tell you about the conditions the animal was raised in and may be able to get you specialty cuts if you are interested. You will also be getting meat that is fresher while supporting your local economy.

One of the best ways to figure out how to choose your proteins is to understand the labels that are often applied to meat, poultry, and eggs. Here, you'll find descriptions of what those labels mean.

ANIMAL WELFARE APPROVED; CERTIFIED HUMANE. Both of these labels have to do with the living conditions of the animals as they are being raised and both prohibit the use of non-therapeutic antibiotics and growth hormones.

ANTIBIOTIC FREE; NO ANTIBIOTICS; RAISED WITH-OUT ANTIBIOTICS. These labels mean no antibiotics are used, ever. To ensure accuracy of these claims, look for the USDA seal alongside them.

Antibiotic usage became an issue because of our nutzo food production system. I won't get into all of the ways that our meat production system has gone astray over the past couple of decades, but it directly led to the overuse of antibiotics. Antibiotics are now used on a regular basis in meat production as a means to promote faster growth and to prevent illness. By "on a regular basis," I mean that small amounts of antibiotics are consistently mixed in with the feed of healthy animals. This promotes the development of antibiotic-resistant strains of pathogens that endanger humans and animals alike.

Purchasing meat that has been produced without the excessive use of antibiotics helps to incentivize the meat industry to curtail this dangerous practice. Look for the label "antibiotic free" to make sure that the animal your meat came from was not given antibiotics during its life.

CAGE FREE. This claim is seen on poultry meat and eggs. On the meat, it is nearly meaningless, as broiler hens (hens destined to be meat) are typically not caged to begin with. However, on eggs it is more meaningful because the industry standard is for egg hens to be kept in cages for their entire lives. This label tells you nothing about antibiotic usage.

CERTIFIED ORGANIC. Just as with all other foods, meats can be produced organically or conventionally. Meat is raised organically when hormone and antibiotic use is prohibited, the animal's feed is 100 percent organic (free of hormones and animal byproducts), ruminants like cows and sheep have at least a 30 percent grass-fed diet, the animals are allowed access to the outdoors, and they are provided with bedding materials.

Those are all good things, for sure. Though organic credentialing does not eliminate all of the problems with meat production, it certainly reduces them. Nutritionally, meat, eggs, and milk from organically raised animals typically have a more desirable fat profile. If you are able to afford it, organic is the way to go.

FREE RANGE. This label is meaningful for animal welfare purposes. It means that the animal is allowed some unspecified access to the outdoors.

GRASS FED. This label applies to meat from ruminants like cows, sheep, and goats and means that the entirety of their diet came from grass and forage. This label has no bearing on hormone or antibiotic usage, though it does specify that the animals must be given access to grazeable land during their growing season.

NATURAL; ALL NATURAL. This label means almost nothing and is not regulated in any meaningful way. Ignore it.

NO (ADDED) HORMONES; RBGH FREE; (R)BST FREE. This label has to do with added growth hormones that are routinely given to meat or dairy cows to speed growth or increase production. You will most often see these claims on dairy products like milk, cheese, and yogurt. While it tells you that hormones were not added, this does not tell you anything about whether the product was genetically modified or organically produced.

LOCALLY GROWN. Because all of the fancy labels we have discussed so far require fees from the producers, local farmers may not be able to afford them even if the meat is raised according to the principles behind the labels. It is a good idea to chat with the vendors at the farmers market and get to know their practices as best you can. Some will even allow you to tour their farms.

Without further ado, let's talk about food.

VEGETABLES TO EAT

There is a wide range of vegetables available to you when following the Ketogenic Mediterranean Diet. In fact, all vegetables can fit into this plan in moderation. However, starchy vegetables like potatoes, sweet potatoes, peas, carrots, corn, and most beans will use up your carbohydrate allotment for the day rather quickly, so they need to be omitted or highly restricted. Nearly all other vegetables can and should be enjoyed liberally. The United States Department of Agriculture (USDA) maintains a list of nutrient values of a huge variety of foods, which is very useful when evaluating what to eat. Remember, you determine net carbohydrate content of a food with a simple formula:

Total Carbohydrate – Fiber = Net Carbohydrate

Here is an abbreviated list of vegetables and their corresponding carbohydrate contents.

VEGETABLE	SERVING SIZE	NET CARBS
Alfalfa sprouts	½ cup	0.2 gram
Artichoke (hearts)	4 pieces	2 grams
Artichoke (whole)	1 whole	6.9 grams
Asparagus (steamed)	4 spears	1.6 grams
Bean sprouts	½ cup	2.1 grams
Bok choy	½ cup	0.2 gram
Broccoli florets	½ cup	0.8 gram
Broccoli rabe	½ cup	2 grams
Broccolini	½ cup	6.7 grams
Brussels sprouts (steamed)	½ cup	4.7 grams
Cabbage (green, raw)	½ cup	1.1 grams
Cabbage (green, steamed)	½ cup	1.6 grams
Cabbage (red, raw)	½ cup	1.4 grams
Cabbage (savoy, steamed)	½ cup	1.9 grams
Carrot (raw)	1 large	6.5 grams
Carrot (steamed)	1 large	5.6 grams
Cauliflower (raw)	½ cup	1.4 grams
Cauliflower (steamed)	½ cup	0.9 gram
Celery (raw)	1 stem	3 grams
Collard greens	½ cup	2 grams
Cucumber (raw)	½ cup	1 gram
Eggplant (broiled)	½ cup	2.1 grams
Endive	½ cup	0.2 gram
Fennel (fresh)	½ cup	1.8 grams
Garlic (fresh)	1 clove	0.9 gram
Green beans (steamed)	½ cup	2.9 grams
Jicama (raw)	½ cup	2.5 grams
Kale (steamed)	½ cup	2.1 grams
Lettuce (Boston Bibb)	½ cup	0.4 gram
Lettuce (Iceberg)	½ cup	0.2 gram
Lettuce (Romaine)	½ cup	0.2 gram
Mushroom (button)	½ cup	1.4 grams

VEGETABLE	SERVING SIZE	NET CARBS
Mushroom (portobello)	4 ounces	4.1 grams
Mushroom (shiitake, cooked)	½ cup	1.1 grams
Mustard greens	½ cup	0.1 gram
Nopal (grilled)	½ cup	1 gram
Okra (fried)	½ cup	4.8 grams
Okra (steamed)	½ cup	3.8 grams
Onion (chopped)	½ cup	5.5 grams
Parsley (chopped)	½ cup	0.1 gram
Peas (regular)	½ cup	6.5 grams
Peas (snow)	½ cup	3.4 grams
Pepper (green or red bell)	½ cup	3.5 grams
Pepper (jalapeño)	½ cup	1 gram
Pumpkin (boiled)	½ cup	4.6 grams
Pumpkin (canned)	½ cup	4.1 grams
Radicchio	½ cup	0.7 gram
Radishes	10 whole	0.9 gram
Rutabaga	½ cup	5.9 grams
Sauerkraut	½ cup	2.1 grams
Scallions	½ cup	2.4 grams
Spinach (raw)	½ cup	0.1 gram
Spinach (steamed)	½ cup	2.2 grams
Squash (butternut, baked)	½ cup	7.9 grams
Squash (spaghetti)	½ cup	7.8 grams
Squash (summer)	½ cup	1.3 grams
Squash (zucchini, steamed)	½ cup	1.5 grams
Tomatillo	½ cup	2.6 grams
Tomato (cherry)	10 whole	6 grams
Tomato (plum)	1 whole	2.2 grams
Turnip greens (boiled)	½ cup	0.6 gram
Turnips (boiled)	½ cup	2.3 grams
Water chestnuts	½ cup	7 grams
Yellow wax beans	½ cup	2.9 grams

Of course, you will be preparing these vegetables in a way that makes them much more palatable—with fat! Covering with extra virgin olive oil–based salad dressings, sautéing in butter, covering in cream sauces, and stuffing with cheese are all encouraged methods for preparing vegetables included in the Ketogenic Mediterranean Diet. There is also an abundance of ways to incorporate vegetables so they do not feel like a grocery store produce section on your plate. For example, cauliflower can be used to make pizza crust, bread, and sushi.

FRUITS TO EAT

Most fruits are too carbohydrate rich to be included in the Ketogenic Mediterranean Diet. Apples, oranges, bananas, mangos, peaches, plums, and the like must all be excluded or heavily limited. However, there are fruits that we do not often think of as fruits that are wonderful additions to and can even be included as staples of this diet.

Olives, for one, are actually a fruit, and because of their excellent monounsaturated fat and fiber content, should be eaten often and with gusto (though I suppose you don't actually need to eat with gusto, if you don't want to; that won't affect the nutrition content of your meal). Avocados are also a fruit and have a fantastic amount of fat and fiber.

Another category of fruits that is good to include are berries. Almost all berries can be included in small quantities. One ounce (28 grams) of just about any common variety of berry has less than four net grams of carbohydrate. They make excellent desserts, too—when combined with fresh, unsweetened whipped cream or plopped on top of some Greek yogurt, berries are divine.

Here is a list of fruits, along with their corresponding carbohydrate values, that are the easiest to include in this dietary pattern. Again, this data is taken directly from the USDA database.

FRUIT	SERVING SIZE	NET CARBS
Avocado	1 whole, medium	2 grams
Blackberries	½ cup	3.6 grams
Blueberries	¼ cup	4.4 grams
Olives	1 ounce	0.2 gram
Raspberries	½ cup	3.4 grams
Strawberries, halved	½ cup	4.4 grams

FATS TO EAT

Because it is based on the ketogenic diet, the Ketogenic Mediterranean Diet necessarily is mostly fat. Of course, as covered earlier in the book, fat is complicated and there are several different kinds.

When eating a carbohydrate-based diet, fat is prioritized as follows:

1. monounsaturated

2. polyunsaturated

3. saturated

4. trans fat

There should also be an emphasis on the consumption of omega-3 polyunsaturated fats. However, the body has the ability to differentiate between fats and appears to have fuel preferences when fat adapted. Not only does total fat oxidation increase when you are in ketosis, but the rate of saturated fat oxidation increases to a greater extent than that of the other fats. Because of this, your prioritization of fats looks different on the Ketogenic Mediterranean Diet. Monounsaturated fats are still in the top spot and artificial trans fats should still be avoided altogether, but the middle two spots switch. Try to prioritize your fat intake as such:

1. monounsaturated
2. saturated
3. polyunsaturated
4. trans fat

The easiest way to tell the type of fat is by how it behaves and appears when cooled. At lower temperatures, saturated fat will solidify, monounsaturated fat will become cloudy and thicken but remain a liquid, and polyunsaturated fat will remain liquid and clear when cooled. Unfortunately, you will not always be dealing with something that is made up of just one kind of fat. In fact, there is no pure source of any one type of fat in the world. Everything is a mixture of fats.

For example, olive oil, which we typically call monounsaturated, is about 75 percent monounsaturated, 12 percent polyunsaturated, and 15 percent saturated. Butter, which has been vilified as a saturated fat bomb that must be avoided, is actually a little over one fourth monounsaturated fat. Don't worry about that too much, though. If you eat mostly fresh foods, lots of vegetables, and get the majority of your fat from olives, olive oil, nuts and seeds, avocado, and fish, the fat percentages will balance themselves out.

Your main source of monounsaturated fat will be olives and olive oil. Olives need little explanation save that they are available in a few different varieties and are occasionally stuffed with increasingly interesting things, like cheese and garlic. Be adventurous but be careful of the stuffing options, as these will affect the carbohydrate content.

Oil requires a bit of a longer discussion. First off, here's a list of common oils and their respective fat concentrations. New oils are available all the time, so keep an eye out for new ones to try. In general, oils should be fine for the Ketogenic Mediterranean Diet because a pure oil of any type will be all fat. Flavored oils may have additives, so check the ingredients.

OIL	FAT CONSTITUENT PERCENTAGES (from greatest to least)
Avocado	~ 71 mono • 16 poly • 13 saturated
Coconut	~ 90 saturated • 7 mono • 3 poly
Hazelnut	~ 78 mono • 12 poly • 10 saturated
Olive	~ 75 mono • 14 saturated • 11 poly
Peanut	~ 50 mono • 33 poly • 17 saturated
Canola (Rapeseed)	~ 63 mono • 30 poly • 7 saturated
Soy	~ 58 poly • 23 mono • 19 saturated

All of the values in the above table were taken from the USDA database and have been rounded. As you can see, olive oil, avocado oil, and hazelnut oil are all great for our purposes, but all of the oils (aside from soy) have a pretty good breakdown.

There are also a few terms you should be familiar with when shopping for oils. "Virgin" and "extra virgin" are quality indicators. Extra virgin means that the oil is obtained through mechanical means and without the use of solvents, it was processed at a temperature never exceeding 86°F, it contains no additives, and it passed laboratory and taste tests.

Virgin may be of lower quality and may have some taste irregularities.

The terms "refined" and "unrefined" appear most often on coconut oil, and they mean pretty much what you would think: Refined oils are obtained from dried coconut and have been bleached, filtered, and deodorized. It has less flavor but is good for cooking because the refining process makes it more stable. Unrefined oils come from fresh coconut and have not been altered. Unrefined coconut oil is also some-times called virgin, but here "virgin" does not denote the same things as virgin for olive oil. Confusing, right?

To add to the confusion, none of these labels are really regu-lated in the United States. Honestly, buying oils in this country is a bit of a guessing game. High-quality oils should have a very distinct, fresh taste of whatever they are derived from. I advise finding a brand that you like and sticking with it.

You can buy the more refined oils for cooking because they will typically be less flavorful and be able to withstand more heat. The fancier, better-tasting oils are going to be more fragile and will need a bit of pampering. Keep them in a dark and cool place because both heat and light can cause these fats to oxidize, which makes them rancid. Keeping them in the refrigerator is not a terrible idea.

MEDIUM-CHAIN TRIGLYCERIDES. Before we move on to protein, let's talk about coconuts and medium-chain tri-glycerides (MCTs). Most of the fats we eat are composed of long-chain triglycerides and have to be transported to the liver in order to be broken down into smaller chains that we can utilize. Unlike almost all other sources of fat, most of the fatty acids in coconuts are MCTs, which can cross from the small intestine directly into the bloodstream.

Medium-chain triglycerides have been shown to promote fatty acid oxidation and ketosis. Research indicates that while MCTs will not initiate nutritional ketosis, they do strengthen it. This means that coconut oil is a fantastic thing to include in the Ketogenic Mediterranean Diet. Plus, you know, it is delicious.

However, be careful about eating too much at once in the beginning. Medium-chain triglycerides are known to cause gastrointestinal problems like cramping and diarrhea. People typically tolerate MCTs very well, but some will have issues. If you find yourself to be in the latter category, don't miss out on their benefits by cutting them out altogether. Just cut back and introduce them more slowly. You should build tolerance over time.

PROTEIN TO EAT

Protein can come from many sources, and though most Americans think the words "protein" and "meat" are synonyms, this is not the case. Although all types of meats that have not been breaded or covered in some sort of sweet sauce can be included, meat does not need to be your only source of protein. Tofu, tempeh, and other meat alternatives are perfectly acceptable so long as their carbohydrate content is low enough.

Let's start with a look at the different kind of meats and meat substitutes and the issues involved with each. Meat from land animals, including beef, pork, and poultry, are all more or less acceptable under the Ketogenic Mediterranean Diet. Many of the labeling issues that were discussed at the beginning of this chapter apply to these meats and to the other proteins discussed below.

EGGS

When buying eggs, you should pretty much consider the same things as when buying meat, but there's the added confusion surrounding different colored eggshells. Here's the shocking secret about white eggs versus brown eggs: there is no difference! The color of the shell has not been shown to be correlated to the nutritional value of what's inside. The color difference actually comes from the type of chicken that lays the egg. Brown eggs tend to cost more in the store because the chickens that lay brown eggs are usually larger and require more feed.

As I'm sure you guessed, I think it is best to purchase eggs from a small, local source if possible. The eggs that I get from my egg guy (his name is Juan and he has about 20 hens) are richer in flavor and color than those I can find at the store. They are usually a little cheaper, too.

Sometimes you will see claims about the omega-3 fat content on the label of some eggs. These claims are true: those eggs have ALA fatty acid in greater concentrations than traditional eggs. This is achieved by feeding the chickens flaxseed. Especially if you are following the Ketogenic Mediterranean Diet, this additional ALA is not going to make that much of a difference, nutritionally. The additional cost of that type of egg will line the pockets of egg producers and marketers, though. My advice is to save your money and eat more fish.

FISH

Believe it or not, the same antibiotic and organic issues carry over to aquatic-based meat, as well. Fish and shrimp farms are not free of the issues that plague land-based meat production, and they actually have a few more tangles to consider. Farmed salmon, tilapia, and other larger fish are routinely fed antibiotics just like factory-farmed cows, pigs, and chickens. If you look for "wild caught" or go organic, you will be free from that issue.

Heavy metal and pesticide contamination can be a concern for fish on the higher end of the food chain, like albacore tuna. Mercury contamination is of particular concern. The US Environmental Protection Agency (EPA) maintains advisory lists on their website, www.epa.gov, regarding how much of what type of fish they consider to be safe to consume. They even have advisories based on specific location. Unfortunately, these advisories are woefully outdated at the time of this writing. The general advisory is from 2014, and the location-specific advisors are from 2011.

An easier way to avoid the issues with mercury is to eat seafood from lower on the food chain. Sardines and anchovies are wonderfully fatty fish, very affordable, sustainable, and delicious when prepared correctly. I know many of you might categorically disagree with the previous statement, but don't worry. I'll give you a couple of recipes that, if you give them a chance, may change your mind about sardines and anchovies.

But what about everyone's favorite fatty fish, salmon? Well, salmon is not immune to any of the issues discussed above, but thankfully, it is not one of the worst in terms of mercury accumulation. Don't eat salmon every day, but do eat it a couple of times a week if you are so inclined. However, salmon *does* come with its own special and monumental consideration: In late 2015, the AquAdvantage salmon became the first genetically modified animal to be approved for human consumption. Though it is not yet available for purchase, it very well may be soon.

MEAT ALTERNATIVES

Finally, let's spend a moment on meat alternatives. There are a staggering multitude of meat alternatives on the market today. There are even some that bleed, though I'm not sure why you would want to retain that particular trait of meat. All types of tofu will be low enough in carbohydrates to fit the Ketogenic Mediterranean Diet, but almost all of the other options will require a bit more thought. Tempeh, a nutty-tasting fermented soy product, is usually fine, so long as it is made exclusively from soy. However, companies recently have started to introduce versions made from black beans, as well. You'll just have to look at the labels for tempeh. Seitan (pronounced say-tan, though fun to mispronounce as say-ten, as in "Hail say-ten!") is a vegetarian protein product made from wheat. It has too much carbohydrate content to fit within our diet. Avoid seitan.

In addition to these traditional vegetable-derived protein sources, there are literally hundreds of faux burgers, hot dogs, sausages, chicken tenders, and more available for purchase, typically in the frozen section of the grocery store. For this myriad of meat alternatives, you'll just have to read the label to determine if they will fit in your carbohydrate budget for the day. I have seen vegetarian burger patties with zero grams of net carbohydrates, but I have also seen them with 18 grams of net carbohydrate.

NUTS AND SEEDS TO EAT

I suppose nuts and seeds could fit into either the protein or the fat category, but I'm going to give them their own section because they are so useful for the Ketogenic Mediterranean Diet. Nuts and seeds, like fruits and vegetables, can and should be a daily part of your diet, but they are not all created equal and not all of them are easy to fit into your daily carbohydrate allotment. Here's a handy list of commonly found nuts and seeds and the corresponding carbohydrate content of each:

NUT/SEED	SERVING SIZE	NET CARBS
Almonds	1 ounce	3 grams
Brazil nuts	1 ounce	1 gram
Cashews	1 ounce	7 grams
Chestnuts	1 ounce	13 grams
Chia seeds	1 ounce	0 grams
Flaxseeds	1 ounce	0 grams
Hazelnuts	1 ounce	2 grams
Hemp seeds	1 ounce	1 gram
Macadamia nuts	1 ounce	2 grams
Peanuts	1 ounce	3 grams
Pecans	1 ounce	1 gram
Pine nuts	1 ounce	3 grams
Pistachios	1 ounce	5 grams
Pumpkin seeds	1 ounce	1 gram

NUT/SEED	SERVING SIZE	NET CARBS
Sesame seeds	1 ounce	4 grams
Sunflower seeds	1 ounce	4 grams
Walnuts	1 ounce	2 grams

Also similarly to fruits and vegetables, nuts and seeds can be GMOs or non-GMOs, and they can be produced using conventional farming practices or organic farming practices. As with the fruits and vegetables, there is little good evidence that one method is hands-down better than the other. However, organically produced nuts and seeds are the more environmentally friendly choice. While the price of organic products, including nuts and seeds, has become more reasonable as demand for them increases, there is still quite a price differential between conventional and organic.

Over the past few years, most likely spurred by the low-carb and paleo movements, there has been an explosion of nut- and seed-based products and flavor options. You can find everything from raw and unadulterated to roasted, wasabi-flavored almonds at your local grocery store. There are also a whole bunch of nut- and seed-based milks available. And, of course, there are butters, glorious nut and seed butters. As with all processed foods, you've got to look closely at the nutrition label for all of these wonder-nut products. Many of the flavored nuts are sweetened in some way, and unless the milks specify that they are unsweetened, they probably are (much the same way that "tea" in the South really means "sweet tea").

Before moving on, I'd like to briefly discuss a few seed super-stars that you may not have encountered yet. Namely, my three favorites are hemp, chia, and flax. I would not eat any of these straight, the way that you would almonds or sunflower seeds, but they are indispensable for salads, baked goods, and jams. Hemp seeds (and hemp hearts, if you can find them) add a fantastically rich, nutty crunch to yogurt or salads and can be used in place of breadcrumbs for coating things like chicken or tofu to be baked or fried. Chia seeds absorb liquid at a rate of about 4:1 and can make low-carbohydrate jams and puddings. Finally, flaxseeds are best used when ground into a meal and added to almond or coconut flour to give bulk and texture to baked goods.

Additionally, you'll become familiar with sesame seeds and sesame seed butter, which is called tahini. Sesame seeds can be used raw or toasted to add crunch and texture to any number of things, and tahini is a delightfully rich, nutty-tasting butter that can be used by itself as a sauce or as a sauce component. It is also an essential ingredient in the Mediterranean staple, hummus. Chickpeas, also known as garbanzo beans, are the other main ingredient in hummus, which we are better off omitting. You can find hummus with sufficiently few net grams of carbohydrate to be included in the Ketogenic Mediterranean Diet or you can substitute cauliflower for the chickpeas and still have a delicious and versatile dip.

DAIRY TO EAT

Ah, cheese. Cheese is fantastic and thankfully can be a healthy part of your day when following the Ketogenic Mediterranean Diet. There are obviously too many varieties of cheese to get into, but almost all of them have good fat content and are very low in carbohydrates. Steer clear of the cheese (and anything else, really) that touts "low fat!" on its label. Not only is that not what you are looking for in this diet, but low-fat cheese is nasty. It tastes and has the texture of plastic. If you are an American-or-cheddar-cheese-only type of person, you must branch out. Be adventurous, but be wary of processed cheese products, which may have carbohydrate-based additives; cheese spreads; and softer cheeses like cream cheese. All of these tend to be a little higher in carbohydrates.

Yogurt can be included in reasonable quantities if you pick the right kinds. Thankfully, Greek yogurt is one of those right kinds. It has been strained to remove much of the milk sugar and is much thicker and creamier than traditional American yogurt. Icelandic skyr is another variety of strained yogurt that is typically very low in carbohydrate content. Just check the nutrition panel and make sure you can fit the carbohydrate content into your budget. Because of the rise in popularity, many Greek and Icelandic yogurts are now sweetened and flavored. Watch out.

Butter and clarified butter (ghee) fit well within the Ketogenic Mediterranean Diet because they have very little carbohydrate and a favorable fatty acid profile. Though you will want to rely more heavily on olive oil for cooking and seasoning, butter has some applications that olive oil is not appropriate for, like baking desserts.

Dairy milk, however, is not an acceptable drink for this diet. An eight-ounce glass of cow's milk contains 12 grams of carbohydrate. It is not worth it. There are, however, several varieties of unsweetened milk alternatives that will fit the bill. I find unsweetened chocolate almond milk to be rather tasty, and it has somewhere between one and two net grams of carbohydrate per glass.

The biggest shopping consideration for all of these milk-derived dairy products is added hormones. Look for a badge or label that says something like "no rbGH" or "rbST free," which means those products have no recumbent bovine growth hormone or bovine somatotropin. They may also be denoted as bGH or bST. rBST is a hormone given to dairy cows to speed their growth and increase production. These added hormones have been linked to an increased risk of breast, prostate, and endometrial tumors. While the evidence is by no means conclusive, many companies have adopted a "no added hormone policy," and these products are not difficult to find.

HERBS AND SPICES TO USE

Of course, spices are what make Mediterranean food Mediterranean. This diet relies heavily on spices to provide flavor and variety. As far as shopping for spices go, you should consider fresh versus dried, conventional versus GMO, and conventionally produced versus organically produced. The same arguments for and against GMOs and organics apply to spices so I won't go over them again. As far as fresh versus dried, fresh is almost always better for flavor, but almost never for convenience.

In case you are not familiar with all of them, here is an abbreviated list of common spices used in Mediterranean cooking:

- allspice
- anise
- basil
- bay leaves
- caraway
- cardamom
- cilantro
- cinnamon

- cloves
- coriander
- cumin
- fennel
- garlic
- ginger
- nutmeg
- oregano
- paprika
- parsley
- pepper (black, green, red, and white)
- rosemary
- sage
- salt
- tarragon
- thyme
- turmeric

DRINKS TO CONSUME

I know that red wine seems to lead many Mediterranean diet articles on the Internet, but the reality is that water will be your main beverage. As I said earlier, red wine can be included in moderation and may have some health benefits associated with it, but it is not a necessity or even necessarily a mainstay. If you do choose to drink red wine as a part of your Ketogenic Mediterranean lifestyle, limit intake to one to two five-ounce servings per day or less. Aside from the dangers of overconsumption of alcohol, a glass of wine contains about four grams of carbohydrate.

Tea and coffee are fine, so long as they are not sweetened with anything that contains digestible carbohydrates. If you are a sweetened-coffee addict, try adding heavy whipping cream, cardamom, and nutmeg to your morning cup. You will find it to be sweet, flavorful, and Mediterranean.

That's it for what you actually eat, but remember, there is more to this diet than eating. For you to fully realize the benefits of a Mediterranean ketogenic lifestyle, you must incorporate the other aspects of the lifestyle into your day-to-day routine.

CHAPTER 9

Embracing the Lifestyle

Earlier I mentioned that physical activity, cessation of tobacco use, moderate use of alcohol, longer meal times, and a greater sense of community are all associated with the Mediterranean life. In this chapter I will elaborate on these things and mention a couple of other lifestyle factors that I recommend including with the Ketogenic Mediterranean Diet in order to get the most out of it and of life in general.

I believe that the cessation of use of tobacco products and the moderate use of alcohol (meaning no more than one or two servings per day) are pretty self-explanatory, so we'll leave those alone. Physical activity, longer mealtimes, stress management, finding a community you feel included in, and getting more (and better) sleep are the lifestyle aspects that warrant a longer discussion and will be covered in this chapter.

PHYSICAL ACTIVITY

Other than tobacco cessation, regular physical activity is the single best thing you can do for your health. Regularly engaging in moderate to strenuous physical activity is both directly and indirectly associated with every health metric you can think of. It strengthens your bones and reduces the risk of fracture, increases your lung capacity, reduces fat mass while increasing lean body mass, improves concentration and cognition, improves mood and emotional outlook, can alleviate insomnia, and is strongly associated with increased longevity.

I would like to address the idea that physical activity is a weight-loss tool: It is not and *should* not be thought of that way. I understand that I just said regular physical activity can reduce fat mass and increase lean muscle mass, and that is true. What I mean is that you can't reasonably out-exercise a poor diet. You would need to walk for five miles or run for almost an hour just to deal with the caloric load of a single 20-ounce soda. That's not a very good bargain, and it is not realistically sustainable as a means for weight loss.

Even if the math worked out better in our favor for "sweating off the pounds," there is good evidence that indicates that most people unconsciously participate in what are called "compensatory behaviors" after exercise. Compensatory behavior is the term used for eating a little extra after a workout because you are extra hungry, or taking the elevator when you would normally take the stairs because you went for a run that morning. So, get physical every day, but don't do it because you think it will help you lose weight. Do it because it will help you live a longer, happier life.

As far as type and amount of physical activity you should be getting, the World Health Organization (WHO) recommends that adults 18 to 64 years old participate in 150 minutes of moderate-intensity aerobic physical activity or 75 minutes of vigorous-intensity aerobic physical activity per week. Moderate-intensity would be walking at a 15 to 20 minute mile pace, cycling at a 5 to 9 mile per hour pace, mowing the lawn or gardening, yoga, actively playing with children, golfing without a golf cart, Frisbee, Frisbee golf, or many other activities that you could fit into your day. The trick is to be honest with yourself about how often you are participating in these activities and for how long.

WHO also recommends including strength-building physical activity in addition to the 150 minutes of moderate-intensity physical activity per week. Unfortunately, I do not have suggestions for leisure-type activities that build strength, but on the bright side, once you get past the difficulty of building a routine, strength building can become a leisure activity. Weight lifting is not the only way to build lean muscle mass, either. All types of impact activities like running, or any activity that involves vigorous movement like dancing or playing sports, will also build muscle and strengthen bone.

If the idea of getting 150 minutes of physical activity a week seems intimidating to you, try breaking it down into daily increments. 150 divided by 7 is only a little over 21. Surely you could go for a 25-minute walk every day, play with your kids for 25 minutes, or go for a nice bike ride. When you break it down into daily pieces, it does not seem so scary or difficult to fit exercise into your busy day.

Taking that idea even further, you can break your activity into even smaller chunks. Most of us are active and awake for 16 to 18 hours per day. If you are moderately active for 10 minutes three times during those 16 hours, you've hit your goal. Go for a walk around your workplace during lunch. Do a sun salutation yoga routine in the morning. Take a nice after-dinner walk. Have three tiny dance parties throughout the day! What I'm trying to say is that getting a decent amount of physical activity does not have to be as daunting as it sounds, and it will make you feel worlds better.

In addition to all of the other benefits of physical activity, it will also help maintain ketosis. Physical exertion will use up more of the available glucose in your blood and prompt your body to break down fat for fuel. This will produce more ketones. It can also be used as a tool to prevent accidentally falling out of ketosis. If you overdo it on the carb load, a moderate amount of physical activity within two hours of the offending meal can effectively use the glucose from that meal up before it has a chance to stimulate insulin release and inhibit ketone production.

LONGER MEAL TIMES

This may seem like a strange thing for me to spend time discussing—who cares how long you take to eat your meals, right? Surprisingly, there are many benefits to slowing down with your meal preparation and time. To some degree, you will not have a choice if you follow the spirit and recommendations in this book. The Ketogenic Mediterranean Diet requires you to cook more and have a greater sense of connection with your food. Because most convenience foods are carbohydrate heavy and because you should strive to eat as many whole foods as possible, you really just have to cook. There's no way around it.

More leisurely meal times and a greater amount of time spent preparing food will necessarily give you a greater sense of connection with your food and with your body. If you slow down, your body will have time to process the signals indicating that you have had enough food, and this will likely lead to eating a little less. This would be beneficial for our collective waistline for sure, but would also be desirable because eating to the point of satiety instead of to the point of fullness would prevent the heaviness and drowsiness that many of us feel after a meal. It would additionally keep your insulin level more even. There are stretch receptors in the lining of the stomach that induce the release of insulin when activated. These stretch receptors are activated by physical pressure on the inner walls of the stomach. If you give yourself enough time to recognize you've had enough before you physically fill your stomach, these receptors will not be triggered, and you can avoid the additional insulin dump.

Based on a study by the Organization for Economic Cooperation and Development (OECD), Americans spend the least time preparing and consuming food compared to people from the 34 countries studied. According to this study, we spend only 30 minutes per day on meal preparation (fast food, anyone?) and about one hour and 14 minutes per day actually eating. If you assume that the average American is only eating three times per day, that is just under 25 minutes per meal. It takes roughly 15 to 20 minutes for you to become aware of the signals your stomach is sending to your brain indicating that it is full. If your total meal is only 25 minutes long, there is just no way that you could catch these signals before overdoing it.

Finally, increasing the amount of time that you allow for meals will help with the community aspect of this diet, as well. There are few joys in life equal to sharing the pleasure of a good meal with people you love. To once again borrow from food writer Michael Pollan, "The shared meal elevates eating from a mechanical process of fueling the body to a ritual of family and community, from the mere animal biology to an act of culture."

STRESS MANAGEMENT

Just about every health professional touts the benefits of stress reduction and knows the dangers of too much stress. Of course, the difficulty is that our lives are stressful. We as Americans work long hours, often for too little pay. We do not get as much time off from work as people from most other developed countries do and many of us don't use the vacation time we have available to us. When you add in bills, kids, commutes, the modern news cycle, health concerns, and the rest, stress management becomes critical.

Much of what we have already discussed will help you manage the stress in your life. Taking control of your eating habits, learning to cook, enjoying more leisurely meals, and getting adequate physical activity will all produce the nice side effect of lowering the impact of the stressors in your life. Improving your sleep habits and finding some sense of community will, of course, help, as well. All aspects of the Ketogenic Mediterranean Diet should help you more effectively manage your stress level.

There are many different approaches to stress management and what works for one person may or may not work for someone else. Many people manage stress through prayer and religious belief. Others turn to family or friends. It is common to use entertainment in the form of television, movies, and games to unwind and de-stress. I personally find that attempting to practice mindfulness helps me deal with the aspects of my life I find to be stressful. The key is to find something that resonates with you.

COMMUNITY

Carbohydrate restriction is not yet an entirely mainstream pattern of eating. If you think about it, many of the foods we associate with gathering are carbohydrate-based: pizza, beer, chips, and birthday cakes are all carbohydrates. Even the common term for sharing a meal is "breaking bread together." When following the Ketogenic Mediterranean Diet, you will likely be eating in a different way than most of those around you, and that can feel very isolating. Of course, it does not have to be this way.

First off, many of the foods that are low enough in carbohydrates to be included in the Ketogenic Mediterranean Diet are foods that will not be viewed as strange. Secondly, a polite decline of that piece of pizza or cake does not have to be a big deal. Just say that you are trying to change the way that you eat for the better and that you have a difficult relationship with carbohydrates. Tell your friends and family that though you won't partake of the birthday cake, you'd still love to share the happy occasion. If you bring the focus back to the occasion, most people will be happy to forget that you are not eating chips or whatever else is being offered. You can also easily prepare foods that are Ketogenic Mediterranean-friendly and still appeal to people eating carbohydrate-based diets. Invite your friends over for a dinner party and cook a meal using any of the recipes you find in Chapter 10.

If you can talk any of your friends or family into changing their eating and lifestyle habits with you, great! Lifestyle changes are much easier to adhere to if you are doing them with someone. You can support each other and hold each other accountable. If, however, you do not have anyone in your life that is interested in making these changes, there is always the Internet. There are many, many ketogenic websites and forums on the Internet. You can find recipes, books, research studies, or just people to chat with on these sites. I'll include a list of some of the best I have found in Resources on page 167.

SLEEP

According to a 2013 Gallup poll, Americans sleep an average of 6.8 hours per night, which is down more than an hour from 1942 and about 40 percent less than is recommended. Getting an inadequate amount of sleep has all sorts of negative health consequences. We cannot focus as well, we do not have as much energy, we do not metabolize foods as well, our systemic stress hormones are higher, we tend to overeat more throughout the day, and we sometimes develop bad hair. OK, I made up the last one, but all of the rest are supported with good science. Sleep deprivation is such a problem in America that the CDC even acknowledges our collective grogginess to be a public health issue.

How much sleep we need varies between individuals, but the amount generally changes as we age. The National Institutes of Health (NIH) suggests that school-age children need at least ten hours of sleep daily, teens need nine to ten hours, and adults need seven to eight hours. If you have trouble getting enough sleep or find your sleep quality to be less than optimal—for example, if you find yourself waking up in the night or waking up in the morning feeling like you have not rested—there are several tips that can help you get more sleep and improve the quality of the sleep you are getting.

First, it is helpful to understand a little bit more about how sleep works. Humans sleep in cycles that are roughly 90 minutes long, with some variation between individuals. There are four stages of sleep that we cycle through, called Stage One, Stage Two, Stage Three, and rapid eye movement (REM). We progress from Stage One through REM and then start over. Stage One and REM are semi-wakeful while Stages Two and Three are deeper, with Stage Three being thought of as "deep sleep." The closer we are to a deep sleep stage when we are awakened, the groggier we will feel. On the other hand, if we are awakened in an earlier stage, it is more likely that we will feel rested and refreshed.

Because of how these cycles work, it is best to try and sleep in 90-minute increments. The best way to determine when you should go to bed is to pick when you need to be awake and then count backward by multiples of 90. You should shoot for five or six full sleep cycles to feel the most rested. This way, you get either seven and a half or nine hours of sleep, respectively. For example, if you need to get out of bed at 6:30 a.m., you should attempt to be asleep at either 9:30 p.m. or 11:00 p.m. You also need to account for the time it takes you to fall asleep. It takes an average of 14 minutes from the time you lie down and close your eyes to the time you are in Stage One of sleep.

If you, like me, find 14 minutes to be a really silly underestimate (it used to take me anywhere from 30 minutes to 2 hours to fall asleep before I started reading about the science of sleep), there are several easy bedtime tweaks you can perform to make falling asleep easier.

For starters, no more checking Instagram in bed. It is recommended that you actually avoid all screens (TVs, computers, phones, tablets, etc.) for two hours before you want to fall asleep. The particular blue and white wavelengths of light that these devices emit inhibit the release of melatonin, one of the hormones responsible for telling the body it is time for sleep. Electronic reading devices, like the Kindle, only get a pass if they do not emit light. The newer backlit models emit the same sleep-damaging blue-white light.

The habit of checking your phone or watching Netflix right before or even in bed is very hard to break. I found it helpful to move my charger all the way across the room and set my phone so that after a certain time it would silence all notifications, including vibrations, so that I would be less tempted to see what the notification was about.

Related to the above point, be sure your sleeping area is dark. If you want a night light of some kind, purchase one that emits soft amber light. It won't interfere with your hormone levels the same way that blue-white light will. Also, research has found that cooler temperatures are more conducive to good sleep. Somewhere around 65°F appears to be optimal.

If you are sensitive to caffeine, you should also consider avoiding it after about 2 p.m. This is a general recommendation, so you may need to stop earlier or later. Caffeine has an extremely variable effect depending on the individual; it can be metabolized very slowly and may still be exerting an effect many hours after ingestion in susceptible individuals.

The CDC also recommends trying to go to bed at roughly the same time each night, avoiding large meals close to bedtime, and avoiding nicotine. See, quitting smoking can even help you sleep better!

A final piece of advice for making the lasting lifestyle changes that will allow you to get the maximum benefit from the Ketogenic Mediterranean Diet: Make one change at a time. Research indicates that individuals actually have a finite amount of willpower at their disposal and that every day is a zero-sum game. If you spend some willpower on avoiding that sugar-laden latte that you are used to in the morning, you will literally have less willpower to spend on your workout later in the day. Make one change at a time and give it a week or two to become a habit before embarking on your next change.

Now, onto the exciting part: recipes!

CHAPTER 10

Recipes

Of what use is diet and lifestyle book without recipes? The answer is, of course, none. None at all.

Aside from it making you feel better, helping you lose weight, lowering your risk of many chronic diseases, giving you more energy, increasing your mental clarity, and promoting longevity, the Ketogenic Mediterranean Diet is delicious. I'll provide you with enough recipes so that you can actually make a go of it.

The recipes in this chapter are a mixture of recipes that I have created from scratch and ones that I have adapted from traditional Mediterranean dishes. They are separated into breakfast, lunch, dinner, and desserts. I'll also give you some bread recipes that will be utilized in a few of the other recipes.

A word about my naming structure: Because I've done my best to make sure all of these recipes will evoke the Mediterranean when you eat them, I am not going to be calling each one "Mediterranean this thing" or "Mediterranean that thing." If it makes you feel better, you may mentally add the word Mediterranean before any or all of the following recipes.

And finally, unless I say otherwise, when I say salt in these recipes, I mean non-iodized sea salt. I don't think that sea salt carries any particular health benefits; I just don't want you to be getting too much iodine. You should be eating more salt to counter your ketosis-induced electrolyte losses, but most table salt has added iodine and you may be getting too much if you use exclusively table salt. Sea salt will also have iodine, but not as much as the iodized table salt variety.

Breakfast

I know that in a traditional SAD diet, breakfast is really code for "starting the day with dessert," but that is not the case with the Ketogenic Mediterranean Diet. As you lose your addiction to sweets and carbohydrates, having a clear distinction between breakfast foods and everything else will become less important. I'm going to put things that seem like breakfast foods under this heading, but understand that you can do what you want with them. I won't come get you if you eat these recipes for lunch, or eat a dinner recipe for breakfast.

Feta and Mushroom Omelet

For years in my home, "omelet" was code for a curse-word riddled attempt at making an omelet that really came out as scrambled eggs. But honestly, that's just fine. The flavor of the dish will be pretty much the same whether it is a beautiful envelope of egg or a beautiful pile of egg.

I don't know of any magic tricks for effortless and beautiful omelets every time. My years of cursing have yielded these tips, though: make sure your skillet is sufficiently lubricated with either some kind of fat or a non-stick coating to prevent sticking, and allow the eggs to cook enough so that they are pretty firm before attempting a flip.

YIELD: 1 SERVING

The Stuff:

2 tablespoons olive oil

¼ cup chopped onion

1 clove garlic, minced

½ cup sliced mushrooms

3 eggs

1 tablespoon heavy whipping cream

½ teaspoon ground oregano (optional)

¼ cup crumbled feta cheese

salt and pepper, to taste

What to Do:

1 Heat the olive oil in a large skillet over medium heat. Add onions and garlic; cook until onions are translucent. Add mushrooms and continue to cook until mushrooms soften.

2 In a bowl, mix eggs and heavy whipping cream. Pour mixture into skillet. Season with oregano (if using), salt, and pepper. Let cook for about 30 seconds and then begin lifting the edges with a spatula while tilting the pan so uncooked egg flows to the pan's surface. When the egg is nearly set, flip the omelet.

3 Sprinkle cheese evenly over the omelet. Cook for about 30 more seconds, fold, and plate.

Salmon and Cream Cheese Omelet

YIELD: 1 SERVING

The Stuff:

2 tablespoons olive oil

3 eggs

1 tablespoon heavy whipping cream

3 ounces smoked salmon

1 ounce cream cheese

2 scallions, chopped

salt and pepper, to taste

What to Do:

1 Heat the olive oil in a medium skillet over medium heat. In a bowl, whisk the eggs and heavy whipping cream together and pour into the skillet.

2 When the eggs begin to set, add the smoked salmon and cream cheese in chunks across the surface of the omelet. Cook for another 30 seconds to a minute until the eggs are set fully. Add half of the scallions and fold omelet.

3 Plate and garnish with the remaining scallions. Add salt and pepper to taste.

Tomato and Olive Frittata

Frittatas are more or less crustless quiches. They are very easy to get right, but also very easy to get wrong. You want the consistency of a frittata to be much like a custard, so it is important to never overcook a frittata.

YIELD: 1 SERVING

The Stuff:

1 tablespoon olive oil

½ cup asparagus, cut into ¼-inch pieces

¼ cup sliced mushrooms

3 cherry tomatoes, halved

¼ cup heavy whipping cream

3 eggs

1 teaspoon oregano

1 teaspoon chopped fresh parsley

¼ cup sliced Kalamata olives

salt and pepper, to taste

What to Do:

1 Heat the olive oil in a medium cast-iron skillet over medium heat.

2 Add asparagus and mushrooms. Cook until soft, then add the tomatoes and cook for 30 to 40 more seconds.

3 In a bowl, mix heavy whipping cream, eggs, spices, Kalamata olives, salt and pepper. Pour mixture into skillet and stir to ensure even distribution of the other ingredients. Cook for 2 to 3 minutes, until the mixture just begins to set.

4 Place the pan into the oven and broil for an addition minute or two, until the top is light brown and fluffy. Remove from oven, slice into equal portions, and serve immediately. It should be noted that you could eat this entire recipe as a meal if you like. It only has about 600 calories and two net grams of carbohydrate.

TIP: Cast-iron skillets are ideal for frittatas because of how they retain and distribute heat. If you don't have one, you can certainly get by with a different type of oven-safe pan or skillet, but you'll have a harder time achieving the firm, crust-like sides and custard-like innards.

Crustless Mini-Quiche

These crustless mini quiches (or mini frittatas, if you like) are great because they are so convenient to eat and they are great chilled, as well. Eat some straight out of the oven and then put the rest in the fridge, and you've got breakfast covered for several days.

YIELD: 4 (3-QUICHE) SERVINGS

The Stuff:

1 ounce cooking oil

½ cup broccoli florets, chopped into small pieces

2 tablespoons chopped fresh parsley

6 large eggs

½ cup grated Parmesan

½ teaspoon salt

¼ teaspoon pepper

½ cup heavy whipping cream

½ cup shredded Swiss cheese

What to Do:

1 Place racks in upper and lower thirds of oven and preheat to 350°F.

2 Coat a 12-cup muffin tin with cooking oil. Scatter broccoli and parsley over bottom of each cup.

3 Whisk eggs with Parmesan, salt, and pepper in a large bowl. Mix in heavy whipping cream until smooth. Evenly distribute mixture into each cup of the muffin tin. Don't make a mess. Top each cup with a pinch of Swiss cheese.

4 Bake until quiches are puffed and browned on top, about 30 minutes, rotating pans after 15 minutes.

5 Immediately run a small, sharp knife around outside of each quiche, then invert onto a wire rack to cool. Turn each quiche right side up. Don't burn your mouth when you eat one or two before they are properly cooled!

Morning Yogurt Cup

Yogurt is just fantastic. It is creamy, fresh tasting, pretty filling, and very versatile. For this recipe, I'm going to say that you can use any of the many soft cheeses with a yogurt-like consistency, but if you stick with actual yogurt you will be getting the added benefit of live, active cultures. These are great for digestion and help ensure a well-balanced microbiome.

YIELD: 1 SERVING

The Stuff:

½ cup plain Greek yogurt, mascarpone cheese, crème fraiche, English clotted cream, farmers cheese, or other soft cheese

1 tablespoon hemp hearts or chia seeds

1 ounce low-carbohydrate berries

1 ounce low-carbohydrate nuts, chopped

What to Do:

Fold all ingredients together in a bowl. It's that simple!

Sardine and Avocado Toast

I told you that I would be providing you with a few ways to use more sardines in your day-to-day routine. Many people are scared of the potent flavor of sardines and avoid them altogether. This, I contend, is a mistake. Sardines are wonderfully nutritious and, when properly prepared, appropriate for any meal.

I first saw a version of this recipe on the illustrious Alton Brown's television show, *Good Eats*. I've since altered it so it fits my liking and is more ketosis friendly.

YIELD: 1 SERVING

The Stuff:

Quick Keto Bread (page 146)

½ lemon

1 can sardines packed in olive oil (with lemon, if available)

1 teaspoon crushed red pepper flakes

½ ripe avocado

½ teaspoon cilantro

salt and pepper, to taste

What to Do:

1 Slice the Quick Keto Bread in half and toast it in a toaster.

2 Zest and juice the lemon into a mixing bowl. Add the oil from the can of sardines, and crushed red pepper flakes to the bowl to create your marinade.

3 Add the sardines to this mixture and gently break them into half-inch chucks with a fork, making sure to cover with marinade.

4 Extract the flesh from the avocado, mash to desired consistency, and spread on the toast.

5 Top the avocado-covered toast with the sardine chucks, a sprinkle of the remaining marinade, cilantro, salt, and pepper.

Fat Coffee

You may have heard that this recipe, sometimes referred to as "bulletproof coffee," has the ability to burn fat extra hard and give you some sort of magical powers. That's all marketing hype, unfortunately. Coffee with fat in it is delicious and can hold you over until lunchtime or beyond, but that's all it is: coffee with fat in it. Don't fall for the hype and spend extra on branded bulletproof coffee, butter, or anything else with that much nonsense marketing behind it.

YIELD: 1 SERVING

The Stuff:

2 cups strong coffee

½ teaspoon cardamom

½ teaspoon cinnamon

¼ teaspoon salt

2 tablespoons butter

2 tablespoons coconut oil

2 tablespoons heavy whipping cream

What to Do:

Put all ingredients in a blender and blend until frothy and decadent, and drink.

TIP: If you enjoy this recipe and think you'll make it often, I recommend getting an ice tray and freezing your butter and coconut oil into cubes. This makes them easier to handle and provides the added benefit of cooling your coffee down to a reasonable drinking temperature faster.

Lunch

One of the interesting things about carbohydrate restriction and fatty acid metabolism is that many people find themselves needing to eat far less frequently. Some people find that they are not hungry until dinner and don't bother with lunch. However, I am not one of those individuals. Here are some of my favorite go-to lunches.

Grilled Sardines and Avocado

I stumbled upon grilling avocados when trying to justify my impulse purchase of a cast-iron grill pan, and my life hasn't been the same since. Grilling imbues the avocado with a rich, creamy complexity that it does not otherwise have. You can achieve close to the same thing with baking, but without some charring, it is just not exactly right. This recipe can be achieved on a grill, grill appliance, or a grill pan.

YIELD: 1 SERVING

The Stuff:

1 tin sardines packed in olive oil

½ tablespoon crushed red pepper flakes

1 teaspoon garlic powder

1 teaspoon turmeric

1 teaspoon onion powder

1 teaspoon ground black pepper

1 avocado

2 tablespoons ricotta cheese

hot sauce, to taste

What to Do:

1 Drain the oil from the sardines into a mixing bowl. Add the crushed red pepper flakes, garlic powder, turmeric, onion powder, and pepper to the oil and mix. Add the sardines into the marinade and coat well, but be gentle so you don't break them up too much. Allow to sit for 10 to 15 minutes.

2 Heat a grill pan to medium heat for 3 to 5 minutes until the pan is heated through. Slice the avocado in half, remove the pit, and carefully extract the flesh with a spoon.

3 Grill the avocado flesh and sardines until visible but light charring occurs along the grill lines. Flip, and allow the other side to cook.

4 Transfer the sardines and avocado to a plate, add the tablespoon of ricotta to the avocado, and drizzle with hot sauce of choice.

Cauliflower Hummus

Few things say "Mediterranean" like hummus. However, because chick-peas provide a few too many grams of carbohydrates for us to include a lot of traditionally prepared hummus in the Ketogenic Mediterranean Diet, cauliflower comes to the rescue! You can customize this recipe however you choose. Add olives, roasted red peppers, Sriracha, or anything else you like.2 tbsp

YIELD: 4 (½-CUP) SERVINGS

The Stuff:

1 medium head cauliflower

1 clove garlic

⅓ cup tahini

1 tablespoon lemon juice

3 tablespoons extra virgin olive oil, divided

salt and pepper, to taste

water (optional)

What to Do:

1 Preheat oven to 400°F. Oil a rimmed baking pan.

2 Break the cauliflower into florets and toss them in 1 table-spoon of olive oil. Place florets in a single layer on baking pan.

3 Roast for 40 minutes, stirring halfway through to ensure even cooking and browning. Remove from the oven and allow to cool.

4 Combine roasted cauliflower, garlic, tahini, lemon juice, 1 tablespoon extra virgin olive oil, salt, and pepper in a food processor and blend until desired consistency is achieved. If you want it to be a little chunky, blend less. If you would like it to be smoother and thinner, add a little bit of water before you blend.

5 Once you are pleased with the consistency, transfer to a serving or storage dish and drizzle the remaining olive oil on top.

TIP: You can use this hummus in a variety of ways. Eat it with sliced cucumber, sliced red pepper, even pork rinds; use it as a spread on your next sandwich; add a dollop to a salad. Really, go crazy.

Tofu Scramble

Tofu scramble is one of the amazing things I picked up during my time as a vegan; another is the mayonnaise replacement Vegenaise, which I find much tastier than regular mayonnaise. I found the scramble to be so sensational that I continue to make it regularly even though I am omnivorous once more. Typically, vegans and vegetarians will try to sell it as a replacement for scrambled eggs. It is not: this dish does not need to stand on the shoulders of the culinary mainstay of scrambled eggs. Tofu scramble is a delicious powerhouse unto itself.

YIELD: 2 (½-CUP) SERVINGS

The Stuff:

1 package extra-firm tofu

2 tablespoons olive oil

1 teaspoon turmeric

1 teaspoon ground cumin

½ teaspoon smoked paprika

½ teaspoon coarse salt

1 teaspoon ground black pepper

2 cloves garlic, diced

2 tablespoons water

2 tablespoons nutritional yeast

1 tablespoon fresh sage, julienned

2 tablespoons fresh basil, julienned

1 tablespoon fresh rosemary, finely chopped

1 scallion, diced

1 avocado, sliced (optional)

2 slices bacon (optional)

What to Do:

1 Drain the tofu, wrap it tightly in a towel, and put something heavy on it. You're looking to get as much of the moisture out as possible, so a heavy cutting board or cast-iron skillet would work well as a weight. Let it drain for about an hour. If the towel is pretty wet halfway through, change it out with a fresh one.

2 Remove the tofu from the torture device and slice into half-inch cubes.

3 Heat the oil in a skillet over medium heat. While it is heating, mix the turmeric, cumin, paprika, salt, pepper, garlic, and water in small bowl and set aside.

4 Fry the tofu in the skillet, stirring frequently until all sides are lightly browned. Add the spice and water slurry and stir to coat. After the tofu and spices are well combined, add in the nutritional yeast. Cook until sauce achieves a sticky, paste-like consistency; add water as needed to thin out sauce.

5 Remove the pan from heat and add in the sage, basil, rosemary, and scallion, stirring to combine. Allow to cook with the residual heat of the pan for about a minute, and then transfer to a serving or storage vessel.

TIP: Since tofu is mostly protein (low carbohydrate and low fat), you may want to serve this with some avocado slices or bacon. You can also use a plop of this tofu scramble on a salad with a fat-rich dressing.

Basil and Avocado Grilled Cheese Sandwich

This is a slight twist on a much-beloved classic. I'll be using the Quick Keto Bread for this recipe, but you could use any type of acceptable low-carbohydrate bread you come across.

YIELD: 1 SERVING

The Stuff:

½ ounce sharp cheddar cheese

½ ounce Swiss cheese

Quick Keto Bread (page 146)

¼ avocado

1 tablespoon butter

½ tablespoon mayonnaise

several large leaves fresh basil

salt and pepper, to taste

What to Do:

1 Heat skillet over medium-high heat for 2 minutes. While waiting, do your prep work: shred the cheddar cheese, slice the Swiss cheese, slice the Quick Keto Bread in half, and slice the avocado flesh into thin fingers.

2 Put the butter in the skillet and let it melt, then place both pieces of bread in the skillet. After a couple of minutes, flip the bread.

3 Put the shredded cheddar on one slice and the sliced Swiss on the other. After a couple of minutes, while the bread is still in the skillet, spread the mayonnaise on the side with Swiss slices, nestle the avocado slices into the mayonnaise to prevent them from sliding out, and put the basil leaves on the side with the cheddar shreds. Hit both sides with some salt and pepper, assemble the sandwich, and eat as soon as it cools enough for you to hold it.

TIP: You will only be using about one-fourth of an avocado for this sandwich, but don't put the rest to waste! I find that if you leave the pit in the half you will not be using, spritz it with lemon juice, and put it in the refrigerator, it will last a couple of days before browning.

Greek Salad

Again, this is an iconic Mediterranean dish that I would be remiss not to include. As with the hummus, it is very highly customizable and you may make as many substitutions as you like. For me, the non-negotiable aspects of a good Greek salad are an oil-based dressing, Kalamata olives, pepperoncini peppers, and feta cheese. For the dressing, Romano or Parmesan work best.

YIELD: 1 SERVING

The Dressing Stuff:

2 cloves garlic, minced

2 teaspoons dried oregano

1 teaspoon dried rosemary

1 teaspoon salt

1 teaspoon black pepper

1 tablespoon grated cheese

¼ cup lemon juice

1 cup extra virgin olive oil

The Salad Stuff:

½ head of romaine lettuce, torn or sliced into 1-inch chunks

2 pickled pepperoncini peppers

1 slice tomato

½ English cucumber, sliced

½ small green pepper, sliced

¼ small red onion, sliced

¾ cup Kalamata olives

¾ cup crumbled feta cheese

What to Do for Dressing:

Combine all ingredients in a mason jar. Shake like crazy.

What to Do for Salad:

Combine all ingredients in a large bowl. Liberally cover with dressing. Eat like crazy.

Charcuterie Spread

Traditionally a charcuterie is a sampling of cured meats and is often served with cheeses, pickled vegetables, and a bit of nice bread. Our charcuterie is very similar, just minus the bread, of course. I tend to replace the bread with nuts for some added fat. I love a good charcuterie spread when I have more time for lunch because the flavors are often so rich that savoring them is a nearly a requirement.

YIELD: 1 SERVING

The Stuff:

½ ounce hard salami

½ ounce smoked prosciutto

½ ounce smoked salmon

½ ounce Pecorino Romano cheese

½ ounce Brie cheese

½ ounce bleu cheese

1 pickle, sliced

1 ounce olives of choice

1 ounce walnuts

What to Do:

Place all ingredients on plate. Feel fancy and enjoy.

Dinner

Dinner tends to be the most preparation-heavy meal of the day, so these recipes will be a little bit more involved than the breakfast or lunch recipes. Dinner is absolutely the best time to practice those longer meal times that I was talking about earlier. Everyone, following a ketogenic diet or not, can enjoy these recipes. So invite your loved ones over, cook up your favorite of the following recipes, and have a nice, leisurely meal.

Lemon Dill Salmon Fillets

Light, fresh, and buttery, this is my favorite way to prepare salmon fillets. Pair with steamed broccoli or baked asparagus for a great, well-balanced meal.

YIELD: 3 (1-FILLET) SERVINGS

The Stuff:

18 ounces salmon fillets

¼ cup melted butter, plus extra for greasing pan

¼ cup lemon juice

1 tablespoon dried dill

1 teaspoon garlic powder

salt and pepper, to taste

What to Do:

1 Preheat oven to 350°F.

2 Grease a baking dish with butter and put the salmon in the dish. Combine the melted butter and lemon juice. Baste the salmon with this mixture and then season with the dill, garlic powder, salt, and pepper.

3 Bake for roughly 25 minutes until the salmon flakes easily with a fork.

Cauliflower Pizza

In my professional opinion, life is meaningless without pizza. Thankfully, following the Ketogenic Mediterranean Diet does not mean that you have to go without pizza. This is another instance of cauliflower saving the day. This crust is a little heavier and moister than a traditional pizza crust, but also a little extra delicious.

YIELD: 2 (4-SLICE) SERVINGS

The Stuff:

1 head of cauliflower, stalks removed

1 cup shredded mozzarella cheese, divided

¼ cup grated Parmesan cheese

½ teaspoon dried oregano

1 teaspoon salt

¼ teaspoon garlic powder

2 eggs

¼ cup low-carb tomato sauce

3 small marinated artichoke hearts

½ cup olives of your choice

1 Roma tomato, sliced

6 large basil leaves, julienned

What to Do:

1 Break the cauliflower into florets that will fit into a food processor and pulse until you have rice consistency. Put the riced cauliflower into a microwave-safe bowl and microwave for 10 minutes. Let cool for about 20 minutes before beginning next step.

2 After the cauliflower is cool, preheat the oven to 400°F.

3 Line a large bowl with a kitchen towel. Dump the cauliflower rice into the towel and twist it up tightly to drain as much fluid as you possibly can from the cauliflower. I usually go through three or four towels and get at least 2 cups of fluid out before I am satisfied.

4 Once you drain the cauliflower the best you can, combine in a bowl with ½ cup mozzarella, Parmesan, oregano,

salt, garlic powder, and eggs and mix it all up until you get a doughy consistency. Flatten this dough onto a parchment-lined baking sheet and shape it into a circle or rectangle, depending on your preference. Bake for 20 minutes.

5 Take the pan out of the oven and add your tomato sauce, remaining mozzarella cheese, artichoke hearts, olives, and tomato slices, then return it to the oven for another 10 minutes or so. Sprinkle the basil on top after removing the pizza from the oven.

6 This pizza is very filling and you will likely have leftovers. You're welcome.

Tomato Basil Zucchini Pasta

Because you must omit grains and grain-derived products like bread and pasta from the Ketogenic Mediterranean Diet, pasta replacements are useful. Spiralizing zucchini is one option that allows you to add more vegetables into your meals.

YIELD: 2 (⅔-CUP) SERVINGS

The Stuff:

1 zucchini, spiralized or thinly sliced

1 tomato, diced

¼ white onion, diced

¼ cup fresh basil, julienned

¼ cup extra virgin olive oil

¼ cup pine nuts

salt and pepper, to taste

What to Do:

1 Combine all ingredients in a large bowl and toss to combine.

2 Zucchini noodles do not keep very well, so you will need to eat them all within a day or two of making them. It's not hard; they are delicious.

TIP: You can technically slice zucchini thin enough to become pasta with a knife, but it is tedious. I recommend picking up a kitchen utensil called a spiralizer, which does exactly what it sounds like it would do. It is indispensable for turning zucchini or cucumber into noodles, and thanks to an "As Seen on TV" version that hit the market a couple of years ago, they are very inexpensive.

Shirataki noodles are another inexpensive, commercially available option. They are an Asian pasta made from tofu or yam starch that typically have fewer than two grams of net carbohydrate per pound and a mild flavor, making them ideal for absorbing the flavor of sauces and soups.

Artichoke Salad

Artichokes are underappreciated. They are a great source of prebiotic fiber (the type of fiber that aides the microbes in your gut), they are delicious fresh or pickled, and they are decidedly Mediterranean. This salad combines artichoke hearts, a variety of olives, and cheese to make a wonderfully flavorful and filling salad.

YIELD: 8 (½-CUP) SERVINGS

The Dressing Stuff:

2 tablespoons red wine vinegar

1 tablespoon chopped fresh oregano

1 lemon, zested

salt and pepper, to taste

¼ cup extra virgin olive oil

The Salad Stuff:

2 (12-ounce) jars marinated artichoke hearts

¼ cup green olives

¼ cup black olives

¼ cup Kalamata olives

½ green pepper, chopped

¼ red onion, chopped

6 cherry tomatoes, halved

6 ounces feta cheese, crumbled

What to Do:

1 Drain the artichoke hearts.

2 In a mixing bowl, mix together the first four dressing ingredients until well combined. Add the olive oil and stir again.

3 In a separate mixing bowl, combine all salad ingredients expect for the feta. Add the dressing and toss to coat. Fold the feta in until even distributed. Serve.

Chicken Kebabs with Tzatziki

Kebabs! I love things that I can eat off of a stick. This recipe is delicious and gave me the opportunity to provide you with a recipe for tzatziki, a creamy yogurt and cucumber sauce. It is also dead simple. Marinate, grill, and eat!

YIELD: 4 (2-KEBAB) SERVINGS

The Chicken Stuff:

¼ cup olive oil

3 or 4 tablespoons lemon juice

4 teaspoons garlic, minced

4 tablespoons red wine vinegar

1 tablespoon dressing from Greek Salad (page 132)

2 pounds boneless skinless chicken breast, sliced into 1-inch strips

salt and pepper, to taste

The Tzatziki Stuff:

1 medium cucumber, peeled and sliced

2 cups Greek yogurt

4 teaspoons garlic, minced

⅓ cup fresh dill, chopped

1½ tablespoons lemon juice

salt and pepper, to taste

What to Do:

1 Combine olive oil, lemon juice, garlic, vinegar, dressing, salt, and pepper in a bowl and whisk to combine. Put the chicken strips in the bowl and cover with cling wrap. Place bowl in the refrigerator for 30 minutes to an hour.

2 Spread cucumber slices out on a paper towel. Sprinkle generously with salt on both sides and allow to rest for 5 minutes. Wrap cucumber slices in paper towels, squeeze excess liquid out, and transfer to a food processor.

3 Put the remaining tzatziki ingredients into food processor and pulse until smooth and creamy.

4 Heat your grill or cast-iron grill pan over medium heat. Thread chicken onto skewers and discard excess marinade. Cook skewers for 5 to 6 minutes on each side until cooked through.

5 Remove the skewers from heat and drizzle the tzatziki on top.

Creamy Asparagus Soup

My friend first made me this soup as a comfort during a difficult time. As these things go, I now have a hard-wired association with creamy asparagus soup and love. It is creamy and smooth, fresh and lemony, and has a very pleasant salty finish. I hope that it communicates love and comfort to you, as well.

YIELD: 4 (2-CUP) SERVINGS

The Stuff:

2 pounds asparagus

1 medium white onion, chopped

¼ cup salted butter, divided

5½ cups chicken broth

½ cup heavy whipping cream

lemon juice, to taste

salt and pepper, to taste

What to Do:

1 Set aside 10 asparagus stalks.

2 Cut any tough parts from the bottom of the asparagus and slice the remaining parts into ½-inch pieces.

3 Cook the onion and 2 tablespoons of butter in a large heavy pot over medium-low heat until butter is melted and onion is soft. Add the asparagus pieces and continue to cook for about 5 minutes, stirring frequently. Add the broth and bring to a simmer, covered, until the asparagus gets very tender. This should take about 20 minutes.

4 During this 20 minutes of simmering, trim the reserved asparagus stalks in ½-inch pieces and boil in salted water for approximately 4 minutes, until tender. Drain the water and set aside.

5 Remove soup from heat for 5 to 10 minutes. If you have an immersion blender, use it to blend the soup until it is

smooth. If you do not, pour the soup into a regular blender and blend till smooth.

6 Back in the pot, pour in the heavy whipping cream, taste the soup, and add as much salt and pepper as you'd like. Bring soup back to a boil. Once boiling, add the remaining butter. Let it cool enough to taste, add lemon juice to your liking, then add the remaining asparagus pieces for texture.

Bread

Bread is something that most people tell me they miss after ditching their carbohydrate addiction. I understand that. Not only is bread ubiquitous in our food supply, it is delicious and versatile. I won't tell you that the breads that follow are exact replacements for traditional wheat and other grain-based breads, but they are pretty darn close.

The only real limitation of homemade low-carb bread is that it does not keep for very long. Thankfully, all the varieties I have made are so delicious that they get eaten before they have the chance to go bad. You will have to guard these breads from the members of your household that do not follow a ketogenic diet because they *will* try and eat it all.

Almond Butter Bread

This bread is the closest thing to traditional bread that I have been able to come up with. It is fluffy and light with a medium-hard crust and very soft interior. It has a very mild nutty flavor and is very useful for sandwich making. Because of the yogurt and nut butter, it can be excessively moist if it's not well blended or if it's not baked for long enough, so be careful.

YIELD: 5 (2-SLICE) SERVINGS

The Stuff:

¾ cup almond butter

¼ cup peanut oil

3 eggs

¼ cup Greek yogurt

1 tablespoon white vinegar

½ teaspoon baking soda

½ teaspoon salt

butter, for greasing pan

What to Do:

1 Preheat oven to 350°F and grease a bread pan with butter.

2 Blend the almond butter, oil, eggs, and yogurt in a blender or food processor until smooth.

3 Add the rest of the ingredients and give a few more pulses.

4 Pour batter into bread pan and bake for 30 to 35 minutes until golden brown.

TIP: For the best almond butter, I recommend using fresh ground almonds with no other ingredients. If this is not feasible for you, look for a brand with no added sugar. To serve, cuff off a slice while it is still warm and eat it with a pat of butter melting over its steaming goodness; this is just divine. Otherwise, wrap it in a towel and keep it in on the counter for up to three days or in the refrigerator for up to a week. If you would like to make it into a dessert bread, add about a tablespoon of an erythritol-based sweetener and some dried coconut flakes in and on top of the mix.

Quick Keto Bread

To get around the issue of longevity and convenience with low-carb bread, I created a microwavable single-serving recipe that can be made in less than 3 minutes. The flavor and texture of this bread is similar to traditional breads with seed and added fiber, what I call "health bread," in that it has some crunch and a pleasing texture. It is fantastically versatile, as well. You may be unfamiliar with a couple of the ingredients, but I promise they are inexpensive and not hard to find—any larger grocery store will have them.

YIELD: 1 SERVING

The Stuff:

½ teaspoon baking powder

3 tablespoons almond flour

1 tablespoon flaxseed meal

½ tablespoon chia seeds

½ tablespoon nutritional yeast

1 egg

1 tablespoon melted butter

What to Do:

1 Combine all dry ingredients in a small, straight-walled, microwave-safe bowl. The bowl should be deep enough that the dough has room to double in size. Choose a bowl with the circumference you would like your bun to be.

2 Mix the dry ingredients well.

3 Add the melted butter and the egg to the dry ingredients. Mix with a fork until smooth.

4 Microwave the batter for one minute and thirty seconds. Let cool for about a minute; that bowl will be *hot*.

5 Slice the bun in half and use however you like.

Cloud Bread

This bread is, as the name implies, as light and airy as a cloud. It has a very mild flavor and is good to be used as a vehicle for spreads or cheeses. Cloud bread variations are also great for making breadsticks. Add garlic powder and rosemary in the cloud, shape them into sticks, and then sprinkle shredded asiago cheese on top before baking.

YIELD: 5 (2-SLICE) SERVINGS

The Stuff:

3 eggs

3 tablespoons cream cheese

¼ teaspoon erythritol

¼ teaspoon cream of tartar

What to Do:

1 Preheat oven to 300°F.

2 Separate the egg yolks from the whites. If you have a stand mixer, put the egg whites in the mixer bowl and the yolks into a second bowl.

3 Mix the yolks together with the cream cheese and erythritol until smooth.

4 Add the cream of tartar to the egg whites and vigorously beat until they get fluffy and start to form peaks. If using a mixer, use the "high" setting. If mixing by hand, whisk until exhausted.

5 Carefully fold the egg yolk mixture into the firm foam you have just created. You are looking to homogenize the mixture without losing the fluffiness. Fold them together slowly and carefully.

6 Get two cookie sheets and either spray them with oil or line them with wax paper or a silicone mat.

7 With a large spoon, scoop mixture into rounds on your baking pans. You should get about 10 rounds from the mixture.

8 Bake your buns for half an hour. You really have to keep a close eye on these and take them out when they begin to become golden brown.

9 Unlike most other ketosis-friendly breads, you will want to wait to consume these. When they are warm and right out of the oven they are crumbly and brittle like a meringue, because that's basically what they are, but if you let them cool overnight in an airtight container they will become soft and chewy like bread.

Desserts

One of the best things about ketosis is that because your body now runs on fat (which is delicious and can make some amazing desserts) you can make dessert-type items into meals if you want to. Of course you should be eating mostly vegetables so you won't want to do this often, but it is liberating to know that you can occasionally thrive on dessert, if you so choose.

I'll be utilizing erythritol and coconut oil in these recipes, and while both of these ingredients are fine (and in the case of coconut oil, actually quite healthful), they are both also associated with gastrointestinal upset if consumed in excess. Unfortunately I cannot tell you what "excess" means because everyone appears to have a different tolerance level, which could change with exposure. It appears that you can tolerate more of these ingredients the more you are exposed to them, especially coconut oil. So, tread carefully and pay attention to your body.

Cocoa and Cardamom Whipped Cream with Berries

If you've never had fresh whipped cream, you are missing out. It is rich and fluffy in ways that commercial whipped cream can only dream of. Plus, it is more or less all fat, so it is perfect for our purposes. For a sweeter flavor, add powdered erythritol. I personally don't think it needs that, but we're all different.

YIELD: 1 SERVING

The Stuff:

½ cup heavy whipping cream

½ teaspoon cardamom

2 teaspoons unsweetened cocoa powder

¼ cup low-carbohydrate berries

pinch of powdered erythritol (optional)

What to Do:

1 Put heavy whipping cream in the work bowl of stand mixer and mix on high until stiff and fluffy, adding the cardamom, cocoa powder, and erythritol, if using, about halfway through.

2 Put into a bowl, add berries, consume!

TIP: If you have a stand mixer, this recipe is as simple as they get. If you do not have a power mixer you can make whipped cream by hand with a whisk. Just whisk the heavy whipping cream very aggressively until you want to die, and then whip it more until you get the consistency you are looking for.

Peanut Butter Fat Bombs

Fat bombs are a term of endearment for food items that contain a large amount of fat per serving. The Fat Coffee (page 123) recipe would also be considered a fat bomb. In this context, it is used to describe fudge-like concoctions that I find rather difficult to eat at a reasonable pace.

YIELD: 8 (1-PIECE) SERVINGS

The Stuff:

½ cup virgin coconut oil

¼ cup unsweetened peanut butter

liquid stevia, to taste

salt, to taste

What to Do:

1 Put all ingredients in a blender and blend till combined.

2 Pour mixture into mold of some kind—silicone ice trays work well. Refrigerate about an hour, or until solid. Store in the refrigerator and try not to eat all of them in one sitting.

RECIPE VARIATION: There are probably thousands of variations of the fat bomb to be found on the Internet, and you can certainly create your own, as well. They have a very simple formula: two parts liquid fat, one part butter like peanut butter, coconut butter, or dairy butter, flavorings, and a tiny bit of sweetener.

Microwave Chocolate Mug Cake

This recipe is great because we all have those unexpected moments where we *must have chocolate.* Plus, it only takes a few minutes from start to finish. The coconut flour gives this cake an incredibly decadent density that reminds me of pound cake.

YIELD: 1 SERVING

The Stuff:

2 tablespoons butter

1 tablespoon powdered erythritol

2 tablespoons unsweetened cocoa powder

2 teaspoons coconut flour

2 tablespoons almond flour

½ teaspoon baking powder

½ teaspoon salt

¼ teaspoon vanilla extract

1 large egg

What to Do:

1 Put the butter in a large coffee mug or microwave-safe bowl and microwave for 20 to 25 seconds until mostly melted. Add the erythritol and mix.

2 Add the cocoa powder, coconut flour, almond flour, baking powder, salt, and vanilla. Plop the egg on top and mix with a fork until you have a smooth batter.

3 Microwave your batter for 1 minute and 20 seconds. Let cool but not too much because as with traditional cake, it is best fresh. If you want to combine with the Cocoa and Cardamom Whipped Cream (page 150), no one would blame you.

CHAPTER 11

Meal Plan

Hopefully, the recipes contained in the last chapter gave you a better idea of what eating the Ketogenic Mediterranean Diet on a day-to-day basis looks like. It is absolutely sustainable and easy to manage, and you will be eating real foods at every meal. This chapter provides you with a sample meal plan that you can put together for yourself.

As long as you are eating 70 to 80 percent fat, 10 to 20 percent protein, and 5 to 10 percent carbohydrate, you have a lot of freedom in regard to what your meal plans look like. For more meal ideas, the Internet is an amazing resource and there are thousands of fantastic recipes (and some less-than-fantastic ones) available with a quick Google search.

DAY ONE

	MEAL	CALORIES (approx.)	NET CARBS
Breakfast	• Morning Yogurt Cup (page 121) • 2 ounces Brie cheese • 8 to 12 ounces coffee or tea with 2 tablespoons heavy whipping cream	500	6 grams
Lunch	• Greek Salad (page 132)	600	13 grams
Snack	• 1 ounce almonds	160	3 grams
Dinner	• Salmon and Cream Cheese Omelet (page 117) • ¼ cup steamed broccoli with 1 tablespoon olive oil, salt, and pepper	800	4 grams
Dessert	• Peanut Butter Fat Bomb (page 151)	150	1 gram
Total	78 percent fat 14 percent protein 8 percent carbohydrate	2210	27 grams

DAY TWO			
	MEAL	**CALORIES (approx.)**	**NET CARBS**
Breakfast	• Fat Coffee (page 123)	550	0 grams
Lunch	• 1 cup Tofu Scramble (page 128) • Side salad (2 cups lettuce, 5 Kalamata olives, tablespoon crumbled feta cheese, a couple rings of red onion, handful cherry tomatoes, 2 tablespoons extra virgin olive oil, salt, and pepper)	650	9 grams
Snack	• Hard-boiled egg	70	1 gram
Dinner	• 2 Chicken Kebabs with Tzatziki (page 140) • 1 cup zucchini, mushrooms, and onions sautéed in 1 tablespoon olive oil, salt, and pepper, to taste	700	5 grams
Dessert	• ½ cup low-carbohydrate ice cream, commercially available (a few brands exist: Halo Top and So Delicious are the best I have tried)	100	5 grams
Total	78 percent fat 13 percent protein 9 percent carbohydrate	2070	20 grams

DAY THREE

	MEAL	CALORIES (approx.)	NET CARBS
Breakfast	• Feta and Mushroom Omelet (page 116)	700	6 grams
Lunch	• Grilled Sardines and Avocado (page 125)	600	1 gram
Snack	• 2 slices Almond Butter Bread (page 145) • 1 tablespoon butter	330	3 grams
Dinner	• 4 slices Cauliflower Pizza (page 136)	550	16 grams
Total	71 percent fat 19 percent protein 10 percent carbohydrate	2180	26 grams

DAY FOUR

	MEAL	CALORIES (approx.)	NET CARBS
Breakfast	• Sardine and Avocado Toast (page 122)	750	5 grams
Lunch	• Charcuterie Spread (page 133)	530	4 grams
Snack	• Cocoa and Cardamom Whipped Cream with Berries (page 150)	430	4 grams
Dinner	• 6 ounces baked chicken • 2 cups steamed broccoli • 2 tablespoons extra virgin olive oil	470	7 grams
Total	74 percent fat 19 percent protein 7 percent carbohydrate	2180	20 grams

DAY FIVE			
	MEAL	**CALORIES** (approx.)	**NET CARBS**
Breakfast	• 3 Crustless Mini Quiches (page 120) • 8 to 12 ounces coffee or tea with 2 tablespoons heavy whipping cream	470	3 grams
Lunch	• 1½ cups Tomato Basil Zucchini Pasta (page 138) • 2 Cloud Bread breadsticks (page 147)	520	14 grams
Snack	• Caprese salad (1 ounce fresh mozzarella, 1 Roma tomato, fresh basil, extra virgin olive oil drizzle, salt, and pepper)	200	3 grams
Dinner	• Lemon Dill Salmon Fillet (page 135) • 2 cups spinach and ½ tablespoon garlic sautéed in olive oil • 5 ounces red wine	500	7 grams
Dessert	• Peanut Butter Fat Bomb (page 151)	150	1 gram
Total	78 percent fat 14 percent protein 8 percent carbohydrate	1840	28 grams

DAY SIX

	MEAL	CALORIES (approx.)	NET CARBS
Breakfast	• 2 slices Almond Butter Bread (page 145) with a tablespoon butter • 1 ounce Brie Cheese • ½ cup strawberry halves • 8 to 12 ounces coffee or tea with 2 tablespoons heavy whipping cream	600	8 grams
Lunch	• Basil and Avocado Grilled Cheese Sandwich (page 130) • Pickle	700	7 grams
Snack	• 1 ounce macadamia nuts	200	2 grams
Dinner	Restaurant meal: See Chapter 12 for tips on how to make good restaurant choices. I included a restaurant meal to remind you that the Ketogenic Mediterranean Diet is flexible and does not have to preclude going out to eat with friends and family.		
Total	Because of the restaurant meal, I can't give approximate totals for Day 6. Just remember the goals of 70 to 80 percent fat, 10 to 20 percent protein, and 5 to 10 percent carbohydrate.		

DAY SEVEN

	MEAL	CALORIES (approx.)	NET CARBS
Breakfast	• Tomato and Olive Frittata (page 118)	600	2 grams
Lunch	• ½ cup Cauliflower Hummus (page 126) eaten with red bell pepper and cucumber slices • ½ cup Artichoke Salad (page 139)	430	17 grams
Snack	• Microwave Chocolate Mug Cake (page 152)	400	2 grams
Dinner	• 2 cups Creamy Asparagus Soup (page 142) • 6 ounces salmon cooked in butter	630	6 grams
Total	72 percent fat 18 percent protein 10 percent carbohydrate	2060	27 grams

Obviously, your specific needs will vary a great deal depending upon your age, gender, weight, body composition, and activity level. This was only intended to be an example of how to put a week of meals together. For the most part, I left out the drinks because you should primarily be drinking water, but if you want to include non-caloric drinks like diet sodas or flavored waters, you can. However, I recommend trying to wean yourself off of those and stick with water.

I hope you are more comfortable with the idea of embarking on this change and now believe that it is absolutely manageable. Let's move on to tips for eating out on those occasions when you will not have time or energy to cook, or when you want to go out with friends. When those occasions arise, you'll be prepared.

CHAPTER 12

Tips for Eating Out

While it's true that most of your meals should be prepared at home and most of your meals should come from whole foods, the truth is that world that we live in makes it so you will not always have the time or energy to cook—I know I don't! On the occasions that you choose to dine out, there are some things you can do to make the experience less painful for everyone. In fact, with the proper mindset, there is no reason it should be painful at all.

You might expect me to tell you only to eat out at Mediterranean restaurants and then to order only salad or kebabs, right? I know you're not going to eat Mediterranean cuisine all the time, and it is not realistic to expect that. Depending on where you live, you may not even have access to Mediterranean restaurants. There is only one worthwhile Mediterranean restaurant in the city where I live, and I'm not going to eat at that restaurant every time I want to eat out. That would be *really* boring.

I want you to succeed at making this lifestyle change, so I included this chapter to prepare you for all of the situations in which you might find yourself trying to maintain carbohydrate restriction while on the go. The Mediterranean portion of this diet is really more about the lifestyle aspects than it is the food, so although the food is amazing, not everything you eat needs to be Mediterranean inspired. Sticking to the ketogenic portion is much more important. You need to maintain carbohydrate restriction continuously in order to stay in ketosis and to reap the benefits of a ketogenic diet. So while you don't always have to eat Mediterranean food, you must always eat ketosis-friendly food.

I hope you know by now that by carbohydrate restriction and ketosis-friendly food, I mean that you need to limit your total net carbohydrate intake to 20 to 50 grams per day. To do this, you should eat foods that are sufficiently low in net carbohydrates (remember: to find net carbs, subtract fiber from the total carbohydrate content). Now, here are some tips for how to manage this when eating out.

First off, don't assume anything, and ask a lot of questions. Many restaurants will include hidden sources of carbohydrates in their dishes that will surprise you. For example, restaurants will often add milk or even sometimes pancake batter to their scrambled eggs or omelets in order to make them fluffier and make more expensive ingredients, like eggs, go farther.

I find that it is also obnoxiously common for restaurant menus to fail to mention when something is breaded. This can be a real bummer if you order what sounds to be a delicious and ketosis-friendly chicken and vegetable dish only to discover that the chicken breast is breaded and therefore unacceptable. This is why you just have to ask questions:

- Does this have breading on it?

- Do you know if the "spicy garlic sauce" has any sugar or thickener in it?

- What vegetables come in the "mixed spring vegetables"?

- Do your scrambled eggs contain any filler?

- Do you have heavy whipping cream I could put in my coffee?

If the server does not know the answer to your questions, it is best to choose something else rather than risk it. If it turns out that the dish or drink you are interested in *does* contain hidden or unexpected sources of carbohydrate, ask for substitutions. Ask to leave the sauce off, substitute other vegetables, or have a different dressing. Many restaurants are more than happy to make substitutions to better accommodate their customers, though some are not. Again, if the restaurant is not willing to sufficiently alter a dish for you, choose something else. There is almost always *something* on a menu that is ketosis friendly.

When you are asking questions and possibly asking for special treatment, remember a few things:

YOU ARE THE CUSTOMER. You are literally paying to keep this establishment open. It is not unreasonable for you to know what is in your food or to ask for relatively easy modifications.

BE SPECIFIC. The server has not likely read this book or any ketogenic diet book and probably does not know what you are trying to achieve with your questions. If you ask, "Is this low carb?" you and the person you are asking could have very different ideas about what "low carb" means. I've seen items on menus that are labeled as low carb but have over 20 net grams of carbohydrate in them. It is *always* your responsibility to make your needs known and to be specific when communicating those needs. Do not assume that anyone knows what you mean.

BE COURTEOUS. I know that the first suggestion was to remember that you are the customer, but at the same time, remember that you are dealing with humans and that they likely get *a lot* of demanding, and sometimes less than pleasant, customers. If they can't find the information that you are requesting, don't take it personally. If they are not patient with you, be patient with them. You'll have a better day, I promise.

Those are general tips for eating out. Don't assume, especially about the information on menus; be a detective, but a very polite one; and remember that there is always something you can eat. Let's delve a little deeper and talk about the types of restaurants where you are more likely to have an easy time finding something.

GOOD BET RESTAURANTS

Obviously, Mediterranean restaurants are likely to be accommodating. Hummus is not terrible, kebabs are often fine as is, and of course, there is the Mediterranean salad; just be careful of the dressing. Meat cooked on a spit is popular in these restaurants and can fit nicely, but ask if they can give it to you without the pita that it is usually served on. Tzatziki is fine in small quantities.

Mexican cuisine is also relatively easy to adapt. They often have fajitas that are intended to be assembled at the table. If you take away the tortillas, you are left with a meat, pepper, and onion hot salad. It is also very easy to get restaurants to make tacos into salads: instead of meat, cheese, jalapenos, and cilantro on a corn tortilla, you get meat, cheese, jalapenos, and cilantro on a bed of lettuce. Be wary of rice that is not listed as a part of a particular dish and the small strips of tortilla that are often added to salads. Ask questions.

Thai restaurants typically have a robust menu of salads and often have curries that are just fine with no modification, depending on the place and the curry. Make sure to ask what vegetables are included, though, because there are often potatoes in the mix. Asian cuisines of all kinds are likely to utilize tofu as a protein option and sometimes build dishes around it that are fine without modification. Sometimes, you can even convince a restaurant to replace the noodles in a dish with bean sprouts. This makes for a tasty, crunchy, and ketosis-friendly dish.

Indian-inspired places are also very easy. Many of their curry dishes are based on butter, oil, spices, and vegetables, so they do not require any modification. Saag paneer is one of my favorites. It is a delicious blend of spinach, spices, yogurt, and paneer, which is a soft cheese similar to feta. Again, be sure to let them know that you don't need the rice that is likely to come with almost every dish.

American-style restaurants are great because they will usually have a selection of steaks with a choice of vegetables on the side. Easy peasy, as long as you don't order peas, which have too many grams of carbohydrate. Go easy with broccoli, instead.

Seafood restaurants are also good choices. They will have many acceptable items on the menu that require no modification. However, avoid the fried items because they will be breaded.

Breakfast joints are good, too. They often do not have a great selection of vegetables but will usually have tomatoes and occasionally asparagus or avocado. They almost always have a very workable selection of eggs and meats.

WORKABLE RESTAURANTS

While sit-down Chinese restaurants can be good if they have menus that you can order from and dishes that can be modified if needed, buffets are difficult just because you can't possibly know what all of the options contain, and it is going a little far to make the employees walk you through the buffet line and tell you about every item. However, Chinese-style buffet restaurants will often have hibachi grills that will offer cook-to-order items, and there you can get a protein and vegetable grilled up with soy sauce.

Nearly all fast-food-style restaurants will give you a pile of meat and cheese in some form or another. While this option is far less than ideal (you want more vegetables than they offer and frankly, they are gross) it can occasionally work in a pinch if, say, you're on a road trip and don't have any better options.

Sushi restaurants typically don't have much to offer other than sushi. Of course, you can order sashimi, which is very thinly sliced pieces of meat or fish, but it is commonly served with rice and it would likely become prohibitively expensive to get the quantity required to be filling without the rice. Though you may never know; if you ask, they may make you a sashimi and seaweed salad.

DIFFICULT OR UNTENABLE RESTAURANTS

Café-style restaurants that are mainly coffee shops usually only have bakery options, which are typically bread based. They may occasionally have a quiche or frittata that you can eat the filling from but usually, you are just out of luck at places like this.

Donut shops and bakeries are self-explanatory: don't even bother.

That is all the advice that I have for you on eating out, and functionally the end of *The Ketogenic Mediterranean Diet* book. The next and final section is dedicated to resources that you can pursue if you are interested in learning more. If you made it this far but are not interested in learning more, then you may put the book down. Thank you for taking this journey with me.

Resources

I mentioned a few times that there have been many great books written on the subjects we covered. I'm going to back up those claims in this chapter, which is dedicated to the books and websites that I used to gather information and inspiration for this book. I'll divide it into sections organized by topic.

KETOSIS

The Art and Science of Low Carbohydrate Living: An Expert Guide to Making the Life-Saving Benefits of Carbohydrate Restriction Sustainable and Enjoyable

by Stephen Phinney, MD, and Jeff Volek, RD, PhD

Written by a medical doctor and a dietitian with a PhD in kinesiology (the study of the mechanics of body movement), this book is probably the best on the market for someone interested in understanding the physiological rationale behind the ketogenic diet. It covers mechanisms and provides a large body of evidence in support of carbohydrate restriction. In fact, Drs. Volek and Phinney have published more than 200 research papers on ketosis and its practical applications.

The Ketogenic Diet: The Scientifically Proven Approach to Fast, Healthy Weight Loss

by Kristen Mancinelli, MS, RD

If you are looking for a ketogenic book geared toward weight loss, this is it. Mancinelli gives a great step-by-step explanation for how to get into ketosis and use it as a weight-loss tool. She writes in a very easy-to-understand, informative manner that makes approaching what can be an intimidating diet much less daunting. She even throws in some really tasty recipes.

Good Calories, Bad Calories: : Fats, Carbs, and the Controversial Science of Diet and Health

by Gary Taubes

Taubes was a science journalist most of his career before he became particularly obsessed with the poor quality of nutrition science. This book is an exhaustively researched exploration of the science and politics behind our nation's collective philosophy about healthy eating. It is a very convincing indictment of the "fat is bad" dogma we have been force fed for the past 40 years.

www.eatingacademy.com

This is the personal blog of Peter Attia, MD. I do not know how else to describe him other than brilliant and relentlessly obsessed with pushing the limits of human understanding and performance. He is an endless self-experimenter and writes very long, very detailed, and very informative blog posts about many topics pertinent to the fat debate and to human nutrition. His series on cholesterol is particularly interesting.

www.ruled.me

Mostly full of fantastic recipes, this website can also be a good place to find a thriving community of keto fans, many of whom are teeming with success stories.

www.reddit.com

Reddit is a very popular aggregation website where almost all of the content is user submitted and, for the most part, user regulated. It has thousands of "subreddits," which are niche communities on the site. Just add /r/*whatever* after www.reddit.com and you'll be taken to the front page of that subreddit. Below are all of the various ketogenic subreddits worth exploring.

/r/keto
General keto stuff, mostly weight-loss related.

/r/ketogains
This one is geared toward building muscle.

/r/ketosceince
Just like it sounds! Primary research studies abound.

/r/ketorecipies
Again, self explanatory.

/r/vegetarianketo
Worth a look, but not as active as the others.

/r/xxketo
Specifically for women.

MEDITERRANEAN RESOURCES

www.oldwayspt.org

This website provides an amazing wealth of information about traditional diets and lifestyles. Oldways is a nonprofit food and nutrition education organization promoting, well, the old ways. Their website holds study-derived information relating to the Mediterranean diet, as well as a multitude of recipes.

The Mediterranean Diet Cookbook: A Delicious Alternative for Lifelong Health

by Nancy Harmon Jenkins

In this book, Jenkins means "diet" in the basic sense of the word: what we eat, what we should eat, and what we used to eat, at least if you lived along the shores of the Mediterranean. Spanning the Mediterranean from Spain to France, Italy, and Greece, with side trips to Lebanon, Cyprus, and North Africa, this book offers 92 mouthwatering new dishes plus the latest information about the nutritional benefits of one of the world's healthiest cuisines.

Jerusalem: A Cookbook

by Yotam Ottolenghi and Sami Tamimi

Indispensable for the burgeoning Mediterranean cook, this stunning cookbook offers 120 recipes from the unique cross-cultural perspective of the authors, from inventive vegetable dishes to sweet, rich desserts.

A Mediterranean Feast: The Story of the Birth of the Celebrated Cuisines of the Mediterranean from the Merchants of Venice to the Barbary Corsairs, with More than 500 Recipes

by Clifford A. Wright

This is a beautiful beast of a book that can only be described as a masterwork. Wright covers over one thousand years of history and paints a cohesive picture of how the Mediterranean region has developed in terms of geography, culture, and culinary tradition. The book includes maps of both the contemporary *and* historical Mediterranean regions, a detailed explanation of the foods one would find in a Mediterranean pantry, and over 500 recipes. It even has a phonetic pronunciation key.

DIET-TRACKING APPLICATIONS

It is possible to keep a running tally of your net carbohydrate intake in your head, but in this day and age there is really no reason to do that. The easiest way to track your carbohydrate intake is through the use of a smartphone application. There are many of them on the market that function in very similar ways. Most of them draw their core data from the same USDA database that I have been referencing, but many also allow the addition of information from their user base. This means that sometimes you will find errors and inaccuracies with these apps, so be careful. All of the apps I recommend to you will be Android and iOS compatible. If you use a Blackberry or Windows phone or tablet these apps may not be available on your platform, but something similar will exist.

The premise of all of these apps is the same: You enter your food item either by searching for it in their database or by scanning the food item's barcode, and then you enter the amount you've eaten either by weight or by volume. Then, the app will record calories, fat, protein, and other pertinent information in your daily log. You can set limits you'd like to stay under or goals you'd like to meet. Many of these applications also have premium versions that will track net carbohydrates, and they are usually not very expensive.

Here are the ones that I have personally used and can endorse:

MyFitnessPal
MyNetDiary
Atkins Carb Tracker

All three of those programs are very usable and will make tracking your carbohydrate intake much easier. If you find one that I haven't encountered and it works for you, by all means you should use it. I also recommend investing in a simple kitchen scale to make your tracking more exact. Kitchen scales are also very useful for more precise cooking, and more precision means fewer surprises.

Now armed with the knowledge I've given you in this book plus the wealth of information you can find in these resources, go forth and discover just how delicious healthy and sustainable eating can be!

Conversions

VOLUME CONVERSIONS

US	METRIC
1 tablespoon / ½ fluid ounce	15 milliliters
¼ cup / 2 fluid ounces	60 milliliters
⅓ cup / 3 fluid ounces	90 milliliters
½ cup / 4 fluid ounces	120 milliliters
1 cup / 8 fluid ounces	240 milliliters

WEIGHT CONVERSIONS

US	METRIC
1 ounce	30 grams
⅓ pound	150 grams
1 pound	450 grams

TEMPERATURE CONVERSIONS

FAHRENHEIT (°F)	CELSIUS (°C)
140°F	60°C
150°F	65°C
160°F	70°C
350°F	175°C
375°F	190°C
400°F	200°C
425°F	220°C
450°F	230°C

Index

Acknowledgments

I would like to thank Dr. William Andrew Clark for helping me slowly understand nutritional biochemistry, sometimes against my will; Kristen Mancinelli for giving me the opportunity to write this book; all the fine folks at Ulysses Press for tolerating my constant missing of deadlines; and, of course, my wife, Jaime, for showing me where I fit in this world.

About the Author

Robert Santos-Prowse MS, RDN, is a registered dietitian currently based in east Tennessee. He writes and speaks about nutrition science and the politics that influence its direction and interpretation. He holds a master's degree in clinical nutrition as well as bachelor's degrees in human nutrition and communications. To learn more, visit his website, robertsantosprowse.com.